What You Need to Know about Diabetes

Revised Edition

By

The Staff of
Joslin Diabetes Center

Published by Joslin Diabetes Center, Boston, MA

www.joslin.org

617-309-2400

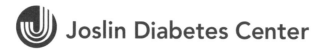

Joslin Diabetes Center

One Joslin Place

Boston, MA 02215

What You Need to Know about Diabetes

Chapter 1
What Is Diabetes?

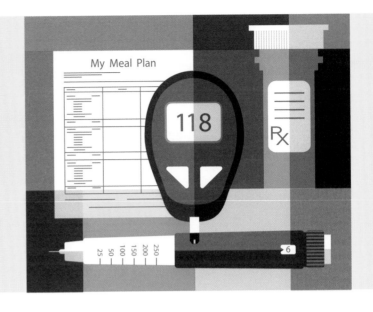

How Your Body Works

It's important to know a few things about how your body works before you can take the best care of your diabetes.

Our bodies change much of the food we eat into a kind of sugar called glucose. The blood then carries this glucose to the millions of cells in the body. When the glucose gets to the cells, insulin helps the glucose enter the cells. The cells then use the glucose for energy or they store it to use later when extra energy is needed. Insulin is a chemical called a hormone, made by the pancreas, which lies behind the lower part of the stomach.

How Diabetes Changes the Way Your Body Works

Diabetes is a disease that occurs when the body is unable to properly use and store glucose. When you have diabetes, glucose builds up in the bloodstream, causing your blood glucose to rise too high, which, if not treated and managed, can cause damage to various parts of the body over time.

Type 1 and Type 2 Diabetes

The two main types of diabetes are type 1 and type 2. In **type 1 diabetes** (which used to be called juvenile-onset or insulin-dependent diabetes), the body completely stops making insulin. People with type 1 diabetes must take daily insulin injections (or use an insulin pump) to survive. This form of diabetes usually develops in children or young adults, but can occur at any age.

In **type 2 diabetes** (which used to be called adult-onset or non-insulin-dependent diabetes) the body produces insulin, but the cells don't respond to insulin the way they should. This is called insulin resistance. In response to this insulin resistance, the pancreas should make more insulin, but in the case of type 2 diabetes, this does not happen. Because of these two problems, insulin resistance and trouble making extra insulin, there is not enough of an insulin effect to move the glucose from the blood into the cells.

Type 2 diabetes is more likely to occur in people who are over the age of 40, overweight, and have a family history of diabetes, although more and more younger people, including adolescents, are developing type 2 diabetes.

High Blood Glucose

When glucose can't get into the cells, it stays in the blood. Too much glucose in the blood is called high blood glucose or hyperglycemia.

You may have symptoms if your blood glucose is too high. The most common symptoms are:

- feeling very tired a lot of the time
- feeling very thirsty and drinking a lot of liquids
- having to go to the bathroom (urinating) often
- feeling very hungry
- losing weight without trying
- blurry vision
- cuts or wounds that are very slow to heal
- frequent infections, such as yeast or urinary tract infections

Short-Term Risks

High blood glucose over the short term increases your chances of getting very sick. For example, people with type 1 diabetes are at risk for a serious condition called diabetic ketoacidosis, or DKA. When the body can't use glucose for energy, it uses stored fat instead. When fat is used for energy, substances called "ketones" build up in the blood and spill into the urine. DKA can make you very sick and must be treated right away. You could go into a coma, or, if it is not treated, you could even die. (Read more about DKA in Chapter 7.)

People with type 2 diabetes are also at risk for getting sick when blood glucose stays very high; however, most people with type 2 diabetes do not develop ketones.

Long-Term Risks

High blood glucose over the long run increases your chances for health problems called *complications*. If your blood glucose remains even somewhat high for many years, research shows that this can increase your risk of damage to your eyes, kidneys, nerves, heart, blood vessels and feet.

> **Blood glucose and A1C levels that are consistently above your target goals may mean that you need a change in your treatment plan.**

Low Blood Glucose

Some people with diabetes will also get low blood glucose. Low blood glucose is sometimes called hypoglycemia or an insulin reaction. If you take insulin or certain types of diabetes pills, you are at risk for having low blood glucose. Just as there are symptoms for high blood glucose, there are certain symptoms for low blood glucose, too, such as:

- feeling shaky, dizzy or sweaty
- feeling hungry
- feeling angry or irritable
- having a headache
- having difficulty focusing or concentrating
- feeling confused

Low blood glucose must be treated right away. If it drops too low, you can fall and hurt yourself, or even pass out. You'll learn more about low blood glucose in Chapters 6 and 7.

It probably sounds like a lot of work to treat high or low glucose and keep your glucose in a safe range. Luckily, there are many ways to help manage your glucose and lower the risk of complications. Here's what you'll learn in this guide:

- how to keep your glucose at a safe level most of the time
- how to take care of high and low glucose levels
- how to lower your chances of developing complications

Symptoms of Diabetes

People with diabetes frequently experience certain symptoms. These include:

- being very thirsty
- having to go to the bathroom very frequently to urinate
- weight loss
- increased hunger
- blurry vision
- skin or yeast infections
- wounds that don't heal
- extreme unexplained fatigue

In some cases, there are no symptoms, this happens at times with type 2 diabetes. In this case, people can live for months, even years, without knowing they have the disease. This form of diabetes comes on so gradually that symptoms may not even be recognized.

Diagnosing Diabetes

If you and your healthcare provider suspect that you have diabetes, you'll most likely get a blood test to be sure. There are three main types of blood tests that will help your provider determine whether you have diabetes. These tests include:

1. *A fasting blood glucose (FBG) test.* For this test, your blood glucose level is checked first thing in the morning after fasting (not eating anything) for at least 8 hours the night before. You may have diabetes if your fasting glucose is 126 mg/dl or higher.

2. *An oral glucose tolerance test (OGTT).* For this test, your blood glucose level is measured before and two hours after drinking a liquid that contains glucose. You may have diabetes if your OGTT result is 200 mg/dl or higher.

3. *An A1C test.* For this test, you will provide a blood sample and from this sample your A1C is checked. The test measures your average blood glucose over the past two to three months. You don't have to fast for this test. You may have diabetes if your A1C is above 6.5%.

Each of the above tests needs to be repeated if the results are high in order to confirm the diagnosis of diabetes.

You may also be diagnosed with diabetes if your random blood glucose is 200 or over AND you have symptoms of diabetes, such as increased thirst, increased urination and/or fatigue. Random blood glucose means the blood is drawn any time of day regardless of when you eat.

The above blood tests must be done in a qualified lab, not at a health fair or by using a blood glucose meter.

How Is Diabetes Treated?

There are certain things that everyone who has diabetes, whether type 1 or type 2, needs to do to be healthy.

They need to:

- Have a meal (eating) plan.
- Become and stay physically active. Activity can help the body use insulin better so it can convert glucose into energy for cells.
- Take insulin injections if they have type 1 diabetes. Some people with type 2 diabetes also need to take insulin or other injectables. Often, people with type 2 diabetes take diabetes pills, which help their bodies produce more insulin and/or better use the insulin it is producing. Some people with type 2 diabetes can control their blood glucose levels with weight loss, a healthy eating plan and exercise, and don't need medication.

Diabetes is treated with:

- A meal plan
- Physical activity
- Medicine

Everyone who has diabetes should be seen at least once every six months by a diabetes specialist (an endocrinologist) or doctor or nurse practitioner. You should also be seen periodically by other members of a diabetes treatment team, including:

- a diabetes nurse educator
- a diabetes dietitian for help in developing a meal plan that works best for you
- an exercise physiologist for help in developing an activity plan
- a social worker, psychologist or other mental health professional, if you think you need it, for help with the stresses and challenges of living with a chronic disease

Everyone who has diabetes should have regular eye exams (once a year) by a specialist in diabetic eye disease to make sure that any eye problems associated with diabetes are caught early, and treated before they become serious.

Also, people with diabetes need to learn how to monitor their blood glucose levels day-to-day at home using home blood glucose monitoring products. This daily checking will help you see how well your meal plan, exercise and medication are working to keep your blood glucose in a normal range.

In the chapters that follow, you will learn in much more detail about how diabetes is treated and what you can do to manage your diabetes.

Remember, YOU CAN LIVE A LONG AND HEALTHY LIFE WITH TYPE 1 OR TYPE 2 DIABETES.

New to Type 2 Diabetes: What to Expect

It can be stressful and upsetting to find out that you have diabetes. This is normal! You will have a lot of questions about what to eat, how to prevent problems and what it means for your future. You may even wonder whether you really have diabetes.

The First Year

The first year after being diagnosed with diabetes may be the hardest time for you. This is because you're just learning what it means to have diabetes and what you can do to stay healthy. What can you expect?

- You will likely be started on a medicine to help control your blood glucose
- You will also need to:
  - learn about nutrition and start on a healthy eating plan
  - get regular physical activity
  - learn how to monitor your blood glucose with a meter
  - have your blood pressure, cholesterol and microalbumin checked regularly
  - get a dilated eye exam
  - check your feet at home on a daily basis
  - reach and stay at a healthy weight

It may seem like a lot, but it gets easier!

The Next Few Years

If you've have had diabetes for more than a year, you've been learning a lot about how to care for your diabetes, and you're likely working on controlling your blood glucose. What should you expect over the next few years? We know that your diabetes will change over time. This is the normal course of type 2 diabetes. Because of this, you'll need, over time, to change your treatment approach.

- Expect that over time your blood glucose levels may begin to increase (this can happen even when you are following your meal plan and being active).
- You may see a rise in blood glucose before breakfast or sometimes 2 hours after a meal. Checking your glucose after meals will help you to see changes in your diabetes more quickly than if you just check it once a day.
- A second or even third medication is often needed to control your blood glucose.
- You might find it harder to lose weight or keep weight off. It may also be harder to stay motivated to continue to eat healthfully and be physically active. Try not to get discouraged. It's very common for people to slip back into old habits. Talking to a dietitian or a diabetes educator, or taking a refresher course on diabetes, can help you get motivated again.

After Ten Years

After ten years, though you've most likely been following your meal plan, getting physical activity and working on controlling your weight, you may be gaining weight. Perhaps you've also noticed that your glucose numbers are going up. What can you expect after having diabetes for ten years or more?

- Blood glucose, blood pressure and cholesterol levels may all be harder to control.

- You may need to start on insulin for your diabetes

- Your eye doctor may tell you there are some changes in the back of your eyes (called retinopathy)

- Your primary care doctor may tell you there is a small amount of protein in your urine.

These changes are common when you have had diabetes for 10 years, and are treatable if caught early.

> About 40% of people with type 2 diabetes start insulin after 10 years.

Chapter 2
Caring for Your Diabetes with Good Nutrition

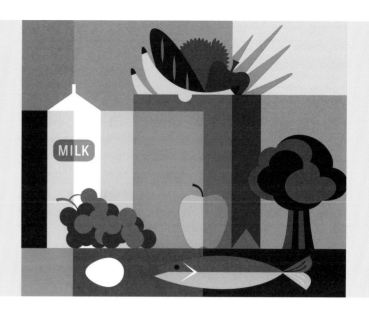

Why Good Nutrition Is Important

Healthy eating is important for everyone. We need food for energy, to build and repair body parts, and to regulate hundreds of processes in the body that help us to function everyday. If you have diabetes, healthy eating is especially important because what, how much and when you eat play a big role in controlling your blood glucose, your weight, your blood pressure and your cholesterol, too.

Eat the Right Amount and Kind of Food and at the Right Time

Your body changes much of the food you eat into blood glucose. The amount of blood glucose that comes from the food you eat is important, especially if you take diabetes medication. The dose of your medication needs to be balanced to match the amount and type of food that you eat each day.

The *amount* of food that you eat is important because:

- If you eat more food than usual, you will have high blood glucose. If you eat too much food, too often, you may gain weight. Weight gain can also lead to high blood glucose.

- If you eat less food than usual, you will not have enough glucose in your blood. If you take insulin or certain types of diabetes pills, your glucose level may go below 70 mg/dl, called low blood glucose.

When you eat is also important, especially if you take diabetes medication. Eating your meals and snacks at about the same time each day helps your diabetes medicine help you. In other words, your medicines help your body use glucose from the food that you eat to create energy or to be stored for use at a later time. Skipping meals or eating meals later than usual may increase your risk for low blood glucose.

How Foods Affect Blood Glucose

There are three main nutrients in food that provide the body with energy in the form of calories. These nutrients are *carbohydrate, protein* and *fat.* Each nutrient has a different effect on blood glucose.

Carbohydrate

Carbohydrate is the body's main energy source. Carbohydrate is like gasoline for your car. Without it, you'll be running on empty, just like a car that has run out of fuel. Carbohydrate is the nutrient that has the most effect on blood glucose. In fact, almost all of the carbohydrate that you eat will turn into blood glucose to be used for energy.

There are *three types of carbohydrate* found in food:

- **starches,** found in bread, pasta, cereal, grains and starchy vegetables
- **sugars,** found in fruits, vegetables, milk and yogurt, and sweets
- **fiber,** found in fruits, vegetables, whole-grain foods, beans, peas and nuts

What foods contain carbohydrates?

- grains, breads, cereals
- starchy vegetables (potatoes, corn, peas, winter squash), legumes and beans
- fruits and fruit juices
- milk, yogurt
- sugar, jam, syrup, cookies, ice cream
- nonstarchy vegetables such as broccoli, lettuce and green beans are so low in carbohydrates and calories that up to one

cup cooked or two cups raw is usually less than 20 calories or 5 grams of carb and are considered "free"

Carbohydrate in foods is measured in grams (g).

> *One carbohydrate serving is the amount of a food that contains 15 grams of carbohydrate.*

One portion of a carbohydrate food that contains 15 grams of carbohydrate is sometimes also called one "carb choice." The Nutrition Facts panel on food labels also lists the total grams of carbohydrate in one serving size of the food. The following are some examples of one carb choice or one serving size:

- 1 slice of bread
- 1 small apple
- 8 ounces of skim milk
- ½ cup of light ice cream

How much carbohydrate do you need?

People with diabetes need to pay special attention to the amount of carbohydrate that they eat. This is because most of the carbohydrate foods one eats turn into blood glucose.

The amount of carbohydrate (or "carb") that you need is based on factors such as how active you are, how old you are, how well your diabetes is doing and the types of foods you like to eat. A registered dietitian can help you figure out the right amount of carbohydrate for you. This is different for everyone. Until you see a dietitian for your own personal meal plan, use the guidelines on the next page to get you started.

Sugar and Sweets

People often believe that sugar causes diabetes, makes you fat or has to be completely cut out from the diet. None of these statements are true. In the past, people with diabetes were told to avoid all sugar, but we now know that sugars and starches act almost the same way on blood glucose, and that sugar added to your meals and snacks, in moderation, can be part of a well-balanced eating plan. The best way to learn how to fit sugar and foods that contain sugar into your meal plan is to meet with a dietitian. Just remember that sugary foods are often high in calories and may contain fat, so it's important to keep portion sizes fairly small.

Fiber

Fiber is actually a type of carbohydrate. But unlike starches and sugars, fiber has practically no effect on blood glucose and contains very few calories. However, we need to include fiber in our diets for good health. Fiber is the part of plants that your body cannot digest. There are two kinds of fiber, soluble and insoluble. Both play an important role in overall health. Aim for between 20 and 35 grams of fiber each day. You can get your fiber by eating several servings of fruits and vegetables each day, as well as including whole-grain foods, legumes, nuts and seeds into your meal plan, too.

- Soluble fiber, found in oats, oat bran, legumes and some fruits and vegetables, can help lower blood cholesterol.

- Fiber can help to slow glucose absorption.

- Insoluble fiber, found in whole-grain breads and cereals, nuts and seeds, can help to prevent constipation and diverticulitis; it adds bulk to stool, keeping stool soft and the bowels moving regularly.

- Both types of fiber help to add a feeling of fullness after a meal, and reduce the need to have snacks. Fiber-rich foods are often low in fat and calories.

- Fiber-rich foods contain special nutrients that may lower the risk of heart disease and some types of cancer.

- Foods that contain fiber have lots of vitamins and minerals that the body needs for overall health.

- Try to choose foods with 3 or more grams of dietary fiber per serving (check the Nutrition facts label on the package).

Protein

We need protein to build muscle and repair body tissue. Protein also gives the body energy, although not as much as carbohydrate does. Protein foods have very little effect on blood glucose, but they still contain calories. Food sources of protein include:

- beef, lamb, pork, veal
- chicken and turkey
- fish and seafood
- eggs
- cheese
- tofu and legumes (beans, peas and lentils)
- nuts, nut butters and seeds
- milk and yogurt

Some protein foods, such as meat, cheese, nuts and seeds, also contain fat. Other protein foods, such as milk, yogurt and beans, contain some carbohydrate. For heart health, choose leaner protein foods whenever possible. Lean meat, poultry without the skin, and seafood that's not breaded and fried are good choices. Aim to keep portion sizes between 3 and 6 ounces per meal (that's about the size of 1 to 2 decks of playing cards).

Fat

Fat is another nutrient that's used as a storage form of energy. Some fats are healthier than others. There are three types of fat found in food: saturated fat, trans fat and unsaturated fat.

- **Saturated fat** is solid at room temperature. This kind of fat can raise blood cholesterol, which then becomes a part of the plaque that builds up in blood vessels. Plaque build-up can lead to heart disease.

- **Trans fat** is a type of fat formed from hydrogenation, a chemical process that changes a liquid oil into a solid fat. Trans fat can increase LDL, the bad cholesterol, while lowering HDL, the good cholesterol.

- **Unsaturated fat** comes mostly from plant foods and is liquid at room temperature. There are two types of unsaturated fat: polyunsaturated fat and monounsaturated fat. Both types of fats are "healthy" and may help to lower blood cholesterol and triglycerides, blood fats.

Fats in Your Foods

The Good	What It Does	Where It's Found
Monounsaturated Fat	Lowers LDL and maybe raises HDL cholesterol	Canola oil, olives, olive oil, peanuts, peanut oil, avocadoes, nuts
Polyunsaturated Fat	Lowers LDL cholesterol	Corn, safflower, sunflower and soybean oils, nuts, seeds
Omega-3 Fatty Acids	Lowers triglycerides (blood fats) and blood pressure	Salmon, mackerel, herring, sardines, flax seed, flaxseed oil, walnuts, soybean oil
The Bad	What It Does	Where It's Found
Saturated Fat	Raises LDL (bad) cholesterol	Butter, shortening, lard, red meat, cheese, whole milk, ice cream, coconut and palm oils
Trans Fat	Raises LDL cholesterol, lowers HDL (good) cholesterol	Fried foods, some stick margarines, some cookies and crackers (look for hydrogenated fat on the ingredient list)
Cholesterol from Food	Too much may raise cholesterol levels	Meat, poultry, seafood, eggs, milk, cheese, yogurt, butter

To lower your risk of heart disease, limit your intake of saturated fat and trans fat as much as possible.

Meal Planning

Plate Method

Eating well can help you control your diabetes and help you achieve a weight that is healthy for you. Until you can see a dietitian to help you with a meal plan, the "plate method" will give you an idea of how much of each food group you should eat at each meal. The plate method is a helpful tool that anyone with diabetes can use. Here's how it works:

- Fill one section of your plate with nonstarchy vegetables: lettuce, broccoli, green beans, spinach, carrots or peppers.

- Fill one section with protein: chicken, turkey, fish, lean meat, eggs or tofu.

- Fill one section with a nutritious carbohydrate food: brown rice, whole-wheat pasta, whole-wheat bread, peas or corn. Choose whole-grain carbs for extra nutrition. Controlling carbs helps you control your blood glucose.

- Include a small piece of fruit at each meal, as well as 8 ounces of lowfat milk or yogurt.

- Add 1-2 teaspoons of a heart-healthy fat, such as olive or canola oil, trans fat-fee margarine, avocado, nuts or seeds.

That's it! Using the plate in this way helps you to eat a variety of foods and helps you easily manage your food portions. This, in turn, will help you control your blood glucose and your weight. It couldn't be easier!

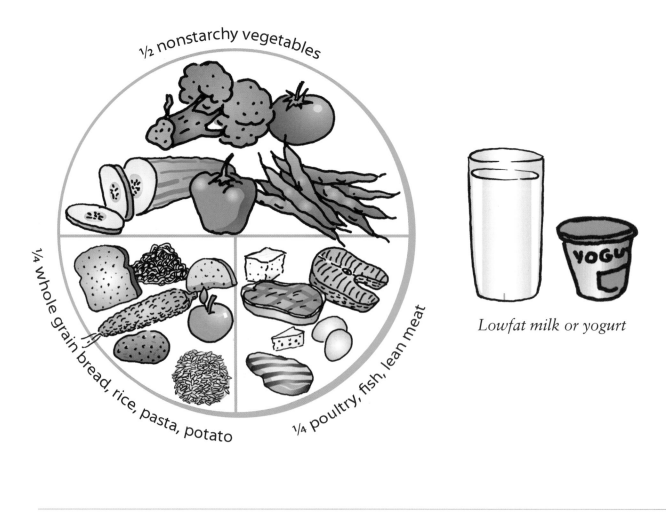

½ nonstarchy vegetables

¼ whole grain bread, rice, pasta, potato

¼ poultry, fish, lean meat

Lowfat milk or yogurt

Your Meal Plan

The plate method and using carb choices are great to get you started. However, you might find it helpful to have a little more guidance with your food choices. You don't need to eat special foods when you have diabetes, but it's important to use a meal plan set up for you by a registered dietitian. Your meal plan will help you keep your blood glucose within your target range, help you achieve and maintain a healthy weight, keep your heart healthy and give you flexibility with your food choices. Meal plans are not meant to overly restrict your food intake or make it hard to manage your diabetes.

All people with diabetes should have their own meal plan that's based on their own goals, the foods they like to eat and their lifestyle. Ask your healthcare provider to help you find a Registered Dietitian and schedule a visit to get your own meal plan.

Your meal plan may look something like the one on this page. Look at the left hand column of the meal plan. The three meals that you eat each day–Breakfast, Lunch and Dinner–are listed in the column. The time of day that you eat each meal is also listed. Notice that the names of three kinds of food are listed under each meal. The three kinds of foods are called food groups, and all foods belong in one or another of these groups. The three groups are:

- **carbohydrate** (milk, vegetable, fruit, bread/starch/sweets)
- **protein**
- **fat**

Look now at the square in the left column where the word "Breakfast" appears. There are numbers beside each food group. If this were your meal plan, the numbers would tell you how many choices of food from each of

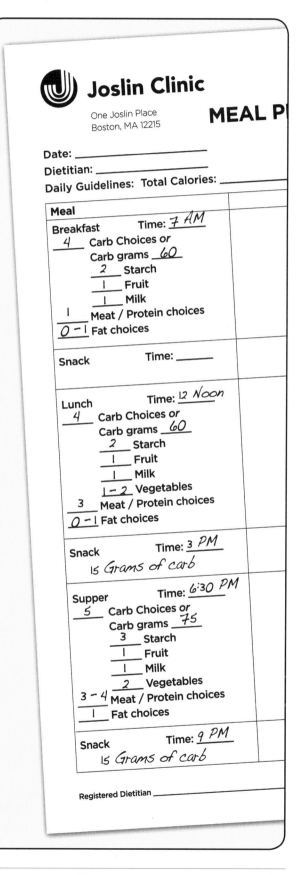

the food groups you may have for breakfast. A "choice" is a certain amount of a food such as 1/2 cup, 2 slices, or 1 ounce.

Using the meal plan on the preceding page as an example, let's look at what you could have for breakfast.

From your carbohydrate (carb) choices:

4 carb choices (60 grams of carb) or

2 starch choices (15 grams of carb each or 30 grams)

1 milk choice (15 grams of carb)

1 fruit choice (15 grams of carb)

From your protein choices:

1 meat/protein choice (1 protein choice)

From your fat choices:

1 fat choice (1 fat choice)

> **All foods can fit into your meal plan, but you need to know how to "count" them.**

Turn now to the Food Choice Lists later in this chapter, or look at the food list your dietitian or healthcare provider has given you. Find the Carbohydrate Group and look under Grains/Breads/Starchy Vegetables. The meal plan you have been looking at lists 2 starch choices for breakfast. If this were your meal plan, you could choose any two foods from this list in the amount listed beside each food. Here's what you might have:

- 1 English muffin
- 1 cup of cooked cereal, such as oatmeal
- 1/2 of an English muffin and 1/2 cup of cooked cereal

If you don't like any of these foods, you could have 2/3 cup of cooked rice or 2 tortillas if you wanted to. Another option is to forgo the starchy foods and choose foods from other carb groups, such as the fruit or milk group. The choice is yours. With meal planning, you decide what you want to eat. All foods can fit into your meal plan. You just need to know a few things:

- what kind of food you want to eat; Is it a carbohydrate, protein or fat food?
- how much you want to eat
- how to "count" that food or fit it into your meal plan

Whole Grain Cereal

Nutrition Facts

Serving Size: 1 cup (53g/1.9 oz.)

Amount Per Serving

Calories 190	**Calories from Fat 25**

	% Daily Value**
Total Fat 3g*	5%
Saturated Fat 0g	0%
Trans Fat 0g	
Cholesterol 0mg	0%
Sodium 95mg	4%
Potassium 300mg	9%
Total Carbohydrate 36g	12%
Dietary Fiber 8g	32%
Soluble Fiber 3g	
Insoluble Fiber 5g	
Sugars 13g	
Protein 9g	32%

Vitamin A 0%	•	Vitamin C 0%	
Calcium 4%	•	Iron 10%	
Phosphorus 10%	•	Magnesium 10%	
Copper 8%			

*Amount in Cereal. One half cup of fat free milk contributes an additional 40 calories, 65mg sodium, 6g total carbohydrates (6g sugars), and 4g protein

** Percent Daily Values are based on a 2,000 calories diet. Your daily values may be higher or lower depending on your calorie needs

	Calories	2,000	2,500
Total Fat	Less Than	65g	80g
Sat. Fat	Less Than	20g	25g
Cholesterol	Less Than	300mg	300mg
Sodium	Less Than	2,400mg	2,400mg
Potassium		3,500mg	3,500mg
Total Carbohydrate		300g	375g
Dietary Fiber		25g	30g
Protein		50g	65g

Calories per gram:
Fat 9 • Carbohydrate 4 • Protein 4

INGREDIENTS: Soy Grits, Hard Red Winter Wheat, Long Grain Brown Rice, Whole Grain Oats, Barley, Rye, Buckwhaet, Sesame Seeds, Evaporated Cane Juice Syrup, Corn Meal, Corn Flour, Soy Protein, Wheat Bran, Oat Flour, Corn Bran, Honey, Natural Flavors, Calcium Carbonate, Salt

CONTAINS SOYBEAN AND WHEAT INGREDIENTS

Reading Food Labels

The Nutrition Facts panel can help you decide what and how much to eat. There is a lot of information on a food label and it can sometimes be confusing to figure out what to look at and what it all means. Use the steps below to make label reading a breeze!

1. Serving Size. Is it more or less than the amount you are planning to eat?

2. Total Carbohydrate. Compared to all other nutrients, carbohydrate raises blood glucose the most. How many grams of carbohydrate do you aim for at each meal? *Remember that one carb choice contains 15 grams of carbohydrate.*

Dietary Fiber can be subtracted from the Total Carbohydrate. Choose foods with at least 3 grams of fiber per serving.

Sugar Alcohols (sorbitol, xylitol, maltitol mannitol) are low-calorie sweeteners commonly used in sugar-free products. Because the carbohydrate in sugar alcohols is not fully absorbed, you can subtract half of the sugar alcohol amount from the Total Carbohydrate. For example, if a serving of food contains 4 grams of sugar alcohol, subtract 2 grams from the Total Carbohydrate.

3. Total Fat and the type of fat you eat should be limited to help control weight and reduce your risk for heart disease. Lowfat foods have no more than 3 grams of fat per serving.

Saturated Fat: Look for less than 1 gram per serving

Trans Fat: Look for 0 grams per serving

4. Sodium tends to be higher in cured luncheon meats, cheeses, canned foods, processed foods and baked goods. Low-sodium products contain less than 140 mg per serving.

Sugar Substitutes

Sugar substitutes are sometimes known as "artificial sweeteners" or "non nutritive sweeteners."

There are six sugar substitutes approved by the Food and Drug Administration (FDA) for use in foods and drinks:

- aspartame: Equal, NutraSweet, Sweet Mate
- saccharin: Sweet N Low, Sugar Twin, Sweet Magic, Sucaryl
- sucralose: Splenda
- acesulfame-K: Sweet One, Sunett
- neotame
- rebiana (rebaudioside A): Truvia, PureVia, Stevia Extract in the Raw

These sweeteners are 100 to 600 times sweeter than regular sugar, so you only need to use very small amounts. Sugar substitutes contain little to no carbohydrate, so they have no effect on blood glucose levels. However, many sweeteners are used in foods and drinks that contain carbohydrate, which, in turn, can affect your blood glucose levels.

> **Sugar-free foods may still contain carbohydrate and calories. Always read the food label.**

Cooking and Baking with Sugar Substitutes

These sweeteners can be used in cooking and baking:

- sucralose
- saccharin
- acesulfame-K
- neotame
- rebiana

Read the instructions on the package for helpful hints.

What Does "Sugar-Free" Mean?

"Sugar-free" means that no white sugar, brown sugar, honey, high-fructose corn syrup or dextrose has been added to the food or drink. "Sugar-free" does not mean "calorie-free" or "carbohydrate-free," because a food may contain sugar naturally, such as the lactose in milk or fructose in fruit.

Read the Nutrition Facts label on a food or drink to decide how to include a sugar-free food into your meal plan. Some foods, such as sugar-free gelatin or sugar-free gum, may be so low in carbohydrate that you can count it as a "free" food. Other foods, such as sugar-free cookies, may have as much carbohydrate as the regular cookie!

Eating Out

You can enjoy eating out and still take care of your diabetes–if you plan ahead.

1. Keep your meal plan in mind. Carry a copy in your purse or wallet.

2. Eat at a place that serves broiled and baked fish, chicken, turkey and small portions of grilled, lean meat. Limit your choices of fatty meats and fried foods.

3. Your diabetes medicines keep working whether you eat on time or not. If you eat later than usual, your blood glucose level may go too low. If you are going to eat a late dinner time eat a small snack at your usual meal.

4. If your protein choice is meat, ask for it to be served with sauce or gravy on the side. Add a side dish of a carb choice such as a small potato or a side dish of pasta, corn, peas or a roll. Make it a point to always include a vegetable and/or green salad for a low calorie source of fiber.

5. Choose a fruit cup or slice of melon if you want something sweet that is lower in carb than typical desserts–or share a dessert with your dining companion.

6. If you are served more food than the amount called for in your meal plan, take the extra home in a "doggie bag."

Healthy choices are available. Plan ahead: If you're going for fast foods, look up fast foods in a book that provides the calorie, carb, fat and protein of specific fast food restaurants or visit the restaurant's Website for nutrition information. A list of some fast-food eating places and some of the foods they serve can be found in the Joslin book, *Staying Healthy with Diabetes: Nutrition and Meal Planning.*

Alcohol

Most people with diabetes can drink alcohol. However, alcohol can cause both high and low blood glucose. If you use alcohol, follow the tips listed below. Your provider will help you keep your blood glucose at a safe level.

1. Check with your healthcare provider or dietitian before using alcohol. There may be reasons why you should not use it at all. If it is okay to use, they will explain how to incorporate it into your meal plan.

2. Drink alcohol only when your blood glucose is within your target range.

3. Cut back on alcohol if you are trying to lose weight.

4. Limit sweet wines, liqueurs and cocktails. They contain carbohydrate that may cause blood glucose levels to rise. Mix alcohol such as gin, rum, whiskey, bourbon, scotch and vodka with water, diet soda, diet tonic water or club soda.

5. Avoid drinking on an empty stomach. Eat some food with your drink.

6. For men, limit the number of drinks to no more than two per day. For women, no more than one drink per day. A "drink" is a 12-ounce beer, 5 ounces of wine, or 1½ ounces of distilled spirits.

7. Check your blood glucose more often than usual if you've had alcohol to learn how it affects your diabetes.

Managing Your Weight

Losing weight is about more than just looking good and feeling better. Losing weight, if you need to, can help you better manage your diabetes, and lower your risk of other diseases and health problems, such as heart disease, high blood pressure, some types of cancer and gallbladder disease.

A large study, called the National Weight Control Registry (NWCR), has been tracking more than 5000 people who have lost a good amount of weight and kept it off for a long time. These people have been able to lose weight, and you can too. The tips below can help you get started with weight loss–and, when you lose weight, help you keep it off!

- **Be confident that you are ready to start.** Your attitude and commitment to success have a lot to do with how successful you will be. If you believe you can lose weight, it is more likely to happen.

- **Diets can work.** The key is to find a "diet," or eating plan, that will work for you. Fad diets may help you lose weight quickly, but you're not likely to keep the weight off for very long. The best "diet" is one that teaches you about making healthy food choices and controlling food portions and that you can follow for a long time.

- **Get support.** You don't have to go it alone. It can be helpful to meet with a registered dietitian for your own personal meal plan. Or try a program, such as Weight Watchers, Jenny Craig or NutriSystem. There are also online programs that can be helpful, including Calorie King and eDiets.

- **Set realistic goals.** You didn't gain all your weight at once, so it's going to take time to lose it. Aim to lose no more than 1 – 2 pounds per week. You're more likely to keep your weight off when you lose it gradually. Also, set a weight goal of losing between 5% and 10% of your body weight. Avoid consuming less than 1200 calories a day if you're a woman, or less than 1500 calories a day if you're a man.

- **Focus on healthy eating habits.** There are no special foods, pills or powders that will make you lose weight quickly. The best way to lose weight is to form new, healthier habits that you can follow for life. Here are some to get you started:

  - Try to eat three meals every day, including breakfast. Eat a snack if you get hungry between meals.

  - Eat plenty of fruits and vegetables.

  - Choose whole-grain foods, such as whole-wheat bread, oatmeal and brown rice.

  - Go for nonfat or lowfat dairy foods, such as skim or 1% milk and fat-free or lowfat yogurt and cottage cheese.

  - Eat more skinless poultry and fish, and limit red meat to no more than 3 times per week. Keep portions to between 3 and 6 ounces.

  - Choose heart-healthy fats, such as olive and canola oil, light tub margarine, and nuts and seeds. But watch portions, because these foods are high in calories.

  - Drink plenty of water.

- **Find ways to be more active.** You'll lose weight more easily and keep it off longer if you include physical activity into your daily routine. Aim for 150 – 200 minutes per week, or at least 30 minutes, 5 times per week. Choose activities that you'll enjoy. Here are some to try:
    - walking the dog
    - using an exercise DVD
    - ballroom or salsa dancing
    - yoga
    - bicycling
    - ice skating or roller skating
    - gardening
- **Monitor your progress.** One way to stick with your plan is to know how you're doing. Here's how to keep track of your progress:
    - keep a food record for at least 3 days each week
    - weigh yourself at least once each week.
- **Wear a pedometer and count your steps**

Healthy Eating Tips

To sum up, here are a few general points to keep in mind when thinking about nutrition and meal planning:

- Eat meals and snacks at about the same time each day. Doing so will help keep your blood glucose more level throughout the day and may also help you to control your hunger.
- Eat about the same amounts of foods, especially carbohydrate foods, each day.
- Choose a wide variety of foods. You need different types of foods to fuel your body and to make sure that you get all the nutrients that you need for good health.
- Cut back on added fat, sugar and salt.
- Aim for a weight that's good for you.

Eating healthfully, reaching and staying at a realistic body weight and being physically active are all important ways to help manage your diabetes, no matter how long you've had diabetes or what type of diabetes you have!

Remember that your healthcare team is your partner in making sure that you stay as healthy as possible. Don't forget that your dietitian is your nutrition partner, helping you to make the right food choices and in the right amounts.

Food Choice Lists for Meal Planning

Knowing how much carbohydrate, protein and fat are in foods can be helpful in planning your meals. Use the list below to help you make healthy food choices. Remember that each food listed is considered to be "one serving" of that food. Your meal plan will tell you how many servings you can have at each of your meals and snacks.

Protein – Meat and Meat Substitutes

0 grams carb, 7 grams protein

Very Lean	Lean	Medium-Fat	High-Fat
1 oz. chicken/turkey (breast, no skin)	1 oz. chicken/turkey (dark meat, no skin)	1 oz. chicken (dark, with skin)	1 oz. cheese (Swiss, American, cheddar)
1 oz. white fish	1 oz. lean beef	1 oz. beef (most products)	1 hot dog
1 oz. tuna (in water)	1 oz. lean pork (tenderloin, ham, Canadian bacon)	1 oz. veal	1 oz. sausage
¼ cup egg substitute		1 oz. feta, mozzarella, string cheese	1 oz. bologna
2 egg whites	1 oz. fish (salmon, swordfish, tuna in oil, drained)	1 egg	2 Tbsp. natural peanut butter
¼ cup non-fat/lowfat cottage cheese		4 oz. (½ cup) tofu	¼ cup nuts

Fat

0 grams carb, 5 grams fat

Monounsaturated (Heart-healthy)	Polyunsaturated (Heart-healthy)	Saturated (NOT Heart-healthy)
1 tsp. canola/olive/peanut oil	1 tsp. regular (1 Tbsp. light) tub or squeeze margarine	1 tsp. stick butter
1½ tsp. peanut butter	1 tsp. corn/safflower/soybean oil	2 Tbsp. sour cream
6 almonds/cashews	1 tsp. regular (1 Tbsp. light) mayonnaise	2 Tbsp. half & half
10 peanuts	1 Tbsp. regular salad dressing	1 Tbsp. cream cheese
2 Tbsp. avocado	1 Tbsp. sunflower/pumpkin seeds	
8 black olives	2 tsp. tahini (sesame paste)	

Carbohydrate Choices – 15 grams carb per serving

Breads, Cereals and Grains	Beans*	Starchy Vegetables	Fruit
1 slice bread (1 oz.) 2 slices low-calorie bread ¼ large bagel (1 oz.) 6" tortilla or pita bread ½ English muffin ½ cup cooked cereal ¾ cup avg. dry cereal ⅓ cup cooked rice/pasta 1 cup soup	½ cup beans, peas (garbanzo, pinto, kidney, white, black-eyed peas) ½ cup lentils ⅓ cup baked beans ½ cup refried beans ⅓ cup hummus *also count as 1 lean meat choice*	½ cup corn ½ cup peas 1 cup winter squash 3 oz. baked potato 2 oz. boiled potato ½ cup mashed potato 2 oz. baked sweet potato ½ cup sweet potato	4 oz. piece of fruit (apple, pear, etc.) 6 oz. fresh peach 6½ oz. orange 1¼ cup watermelon 1¼ cup strawberries 1 cup raspberries ¾ cup black/blueberries ½ grapefruit ½ cup (5½ oz.) mango ½ cup pineapple 1 cup melon 17 grapes 4 oz. banana 12 cherries 1 (3½ oz.) kiwi 2 small tangerines 2 Tbsp. dried fruit ½ cup (4 oz.) juice

Crackers/Snacks	Milk	Desserts/Sweets	
3 cups air-popped popcorn 18–20 mini pretzels 5–8 regular pretzel twists 2–5 whole-grain crackers 3 graham crackers 2 rice cakes, 4" across 9–13 potato chips 9–13 tortilla chips	1 cup milk (fat-free/skim, 1% milk, 2%, whole, lactose-free) 6 oz. light-style yogurt 6 oz. plain yogurt ½ cup evaporated skim milk ⅓ cup dry fat-free milk	1 oz. angel food cake 2" sq. unfrosted cake 1¼" sq. brownie 2 small cookies ½ cup ice cream ¼ cup sorbet 1 frozen fruit bar ½ cup sugar-free pudding 1 Tbsp. jam/jelly 1 Tbsp. honey/sugar	

Non Starchy Vegetables

5 grams carb per serving

1 cup raw vegetables
½ cup cooked vegetables
Non Starchy Vegetables include: lettuce, tomatoes, green beans, carrots, onions, broccoli, cauliflower, spinach, cucumbers, peppers, sprouts, asparagus, artichokes, beets, Brussels sprouts, collard greens, kale, celery, cabbage, Swiss chard, zucchini, summer squash, eggplant, jicama, mushrooms, radishes, mustard greens, and water chestnuts.

Fast Foods/Combination Foods

Casserole (1 cup, e.g. chili with beans, lasagna, mac & cheese	2 carb, 2 protein, 2 fat
Stew (1 cup; meat and vegetables)	1 carb, 1 protein, 0-3 fat
Pot pie (7 oz.)	2 ½ carb, 1 protein, 3 fat
Cheese pizza, thin crust (¼ of a 12-inch pie, 5 oz.)	2 carb, 2 protein, 1½ fat
French fries, fast food (small serving, 2.5 oz.)	2 carb, 2 fat
Burrito with beef and beans (5 oz.)	3 carb, 1 protein, 2 fat
Chicken nuggets (6)	1 carb, 2 protein, 3 fat

Chapter 3

Caring for Your Diabetes with Physical Activity

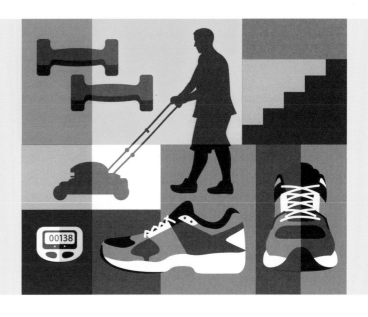

Why Physical Activity Is Important

Physical activity is important for everyone's health, but it is especially important if you have diabetes because of its helpful effect on blood glucose levels. Physical activity lowers blood glucose levels by improving the body's ability to use both glucose and insulin. Many people who take diabetes pills find that they need less medication as they become more active on a regular basis. The same is true for people who take insulin; insulin doses often need to be adjusted to prevent low blood glucose.

Increased physical activity improves your fitness, whether or not you have diabetes, and being fit decreases your risk of all chronic diseases, especially heart disease.

Here's what it can do for you:

- lower your blood pressure
- lower your bad (LDL) cholesterol
- increase your "good" (HDL) cholesterol
- improve the strength of heart, lungs and muscles
- burn off the calories so you can lose weight—and keep it off!
- help you sleep better
- provide an outlet to relieve stresses in your daily life
- help you feel better about yourself

All Physical Activity Counts

"Physical activity" refers to any activities you can do to move your body. Exercise activities like running, using weights or jumping rope are one type of physical activity, but day-to-day activities such as walking, climbing the stairs, cutting the grass, gardening, riding a bike and vacuuming are also physical activity. It all counts!

> **Physical activity is like medicine—but without all the side effects!**

Walking instead of driving, parking the car further away from where you are going, getting off the bus a stop early or taking the stairs instead of the elevator are examples of how you can fit more physical activity into your day. Aim to do something active every day. And choose activities that you enjoy, because you won't stick with an activity that you dislike or that you find boring. Begin by choosing an activity that fits your fitness level and interest, one that you can do on a regular basis. Walking, running, swimming, chair exercises and yoga are some examples.

> **Doing even 10 minutes of activity can help.**

What Is the Best Kind of Physical Activity?

It's important to get different types of physical activity. Aim to include all three in your activity plan.

- *Aerobic exercise* such as brisk walking, swimming, biking or dancing is the best type of activity to improve your stamina and strengthen your heart.

- *Resistance training* helps strengthen your muscles and increase muscle mass. It causes your metabolism to speed up and helps with weight loss. Weight lifting, free weights or resistance bands are great tools to use and reach your goal. Start gradually.

- *Flexibility training* improves the range of motion in your joints. Slow, easy stretches should be done when your muscles are warm, which is at the end of the exercise session.

How Often? How Long?

If you've never had a regular physical activity program before, start off slowly in order to avoid injury. Even doing 5 to 10 minutes can be very beneficial. Then, add a few minutes each week until you reach your goals. If you are already walking or doing some form of regular physical activity, you may be ready to move to the next level.

- *If your goal is to improve blood glucose control and your overall fitness level:* Aim to be active at least 4–5 days a week for 25–30 minutes each day.

- *If your goal is to lose weight:* Aim to be active at least 5 days a week, for 45–60 minutes each day.

Remember, all activity counts! If you can't get all of your exercise in at one time, you can break it into smaller sessions. For example exercising if you are aiming to spend 45 minutes but just don't have that amount of time all at once, try 15 minutes in the morning, 15 minutes in the middle of the day, and 15 minutes at the end of the day.

> Use the "talk test" to see how hard you're exercising.

How Hard?

You should always feel comfortable while doing physical activity. Aim for a pace you can handle — one that is not too hard, but not too easy. The "talk test" can be your guide. You should always be able to talk while exercising; if you can't, you are working too hard. On the other hand, if you can sing, you may not be working hard enough. But regardless, if you do not feel well or feel pain—stop!

Before You Start

Your decision to become more physically active and start a fitness program is an important one. Before you start increasing your physical activity, talk with your healthcare provider. You may need medical evaluations for your heart (such as a stress test), eyes, feet or blood pressure. This is important if you are over 35 years old or have had diabetes for a long time. You may need more information on what is safe and what is NOT safe for you to do.

Take a few minutes to review the checklist below. Mark each statement that is true.

Physical Activity Readiness Questionnaire

(Check each box that describes you):

☐ You have been told you have a heart condition and need to be careful when you are physically active.

☐ You often have pain or pressure in your neck, left shoulder or arm during or after physical activity.

☐ In the last month, you have developed pain or pressure in your neck, left shoulder or arm when you were NOT physically active.

☐ You get dizzy, tend to lose your balance or have passed out.

☐ You have bone or joint problems that get worse when you are physically active.

☐ You take medicine for high blood pressure or a heart condition.

☐ You have a medical condition or physical reason that gets in the way of being physically active.

☐ You're pregnant and your healthcare professional hasn't given you the okay to be physically active.

☐ You are over the age of 35 or you've had diabetes for more than 10 years.

☐ You have type 2 diabetes and are ready to start a new physical activity program.

If you checked off any of these boxes, you can still begin a fitness program. BUT FIRST you need to get medical advice on what you should—or should not—do. Your healthcare provider may want to check out your heart, lungs, blood flow or bone strength. The right fitness program can bring about amazing results; you just need to be safe in your approach.

Lows, Highs and Physical Activity

Your healthcare provider will also help you determine if you are at risk for high or low blood glucose during and after physical activity and, if so, how to prevent it. Generally this is more of an issue for people who have type 1 diabetes, but people with type 2 diabetes who take insulin or certain types of diabetes pills may also be at risk.

How Low Is Too Low?

If you are not taking any diabetes medications at all, but are controlling your diabetes only by changing your eating habits and being more physically active—or if you are not taking one of the medications that can cause a low blood glucose (see Diabetes Medications and the Risk for Low Blood Glucose later in this chapter)— it is not likely that you will have a low blood glucose during or after physical activity. Low blood glucose is defined as blood glucose below 70 mg/dl. The symptoms of low blood glucose are listed below.

Signs and symptoms of low blood glucose

- sweating
- rapid heart rate
- trouble concentrating
- hunger
- feeling tired
- shakiness
- headache
- mood changes

If you use a diabetes pill that may lead to low blood glucose or take insulin, check your blood glucose before exercise. If it is less than 100 mg/dl before physical activity, have a small snack. At the end of your activity, check again. If your glucose reading is under 90 mg/dl, then eat a small snack. *(See the snack suggestions in the table below.)*

Snack Suggestions (15 Grams of Carb)
1 small piece of fresh fruit
2 rice cakes
6 saltines
3 graham cracker squares
1 mini box of raisins
4 ounces of fruit juice
4 glucose tablets
6 ounces of regular soda

Preventing low blood glucose

If you're taking a diabetes medication that puts you at risk for low blood glucose, there are a few ways to lower this risk:

- Plan to be active about 1–2 hours after your meal.
- Eat a small snack that contains carbohydrate before you begin your activity.
- Talk to your provider about changing or cutting back on your diabetes medication.

If you are trying to lose weight, keep in mind that having to eat a snack before you exercise can add unwanted calories!

Diabetes Medications and Risk for Low Blood Glucose (Hypoglycemia)

AT RISK

- Insulin
- glyburide (Diabeta, Micronase, Glynase)
- glipizide (Glucotrol, Glucotrol XL, Glipizide)
- glimepiride (Amaryl)
- repaglinide (Prandin)
- nateglinide (Starlix)
- metformin and glyburide (Glucovance)
- metformin and glipizide (Metaglip)
- repaglinide and metformin (Prandimet)
- pioglitazone and glimepiride (Duetact)

NOT AT RISK*

- metformin (Glucophage, Glucophage XR, Riomet, Fortamet, Glumetza)
- pioglitazone (Actos)
- pioglitazone/metformin (Actoplus met)
- acarbose (Precose)
- miglitol (Glyset)
- saxagliptin (Onglyza)
- saxagliptin/merformin ER (Kombiglyze XR)
- sitagliptin (Januvia)
- sitagliptin/metformin (Janumet)
- sitagliptin/metformin ER (Janumet XR)
- sitagliptin/simvastatin (Juvisync)
- linagliptin (Tradjenta)
- linagliptin/metformin (Jentadueto)
- colesevelam (Welchol)
- bromocriptine (Cycloset)
- exenatide (Byetta)
- exenatide ER (Bydureon)
- liraglutide (Victoza)
- pramlintide (Symlin)

*Note: If you are taking a medication from the "Not at Risk" list along with a medication from the "At Risk" list, you are at risk for having a low blood glucose.

How High Is Too High?

For most people, physical activity lowers blood glucose. Sometimes, though, being active may actually cause blood glucose to go up. There are several reasons why this may happen:

- your blood glucose is too high before the start of activity
- you ate too much food before your activity
- your diabetes medication may need some adjusting

It's important that you check your blood glucose before and after each activity.

- If you have type 1 diabetes and your blood glucose is over 300 OR it is over 250 and you have ketones, **do not exercise.**
- If you have type 2 diabetes and your blood glucose is over 300, **do not exercise.**

Checking your blood glucose is the only way to know the effect of physical activity on your blood glucose.

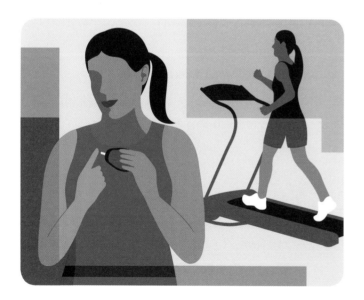

Barriers to Being Active: What Gets in the Way?

If you've never been physically active before, it's understandable that you may have some concerns. Perhaps you've tried to be active in the past and for certain reasons were unable to stick with it, or felt uncomfortable. It's normal to feel this way, but it's just as important to realize that any barrier to being active can be overcome. Here's a list of some of the main things that can get in the way of being active and some suggestions for dealing with them.

Barriers	Suggestions
I'm too busy/I don't have time!	• Make an appointment to exercise mark it on your calendar or in your date book. • Plan your activity at the same time each day to make it part of your daily routine. • Combine activity with another event, such as going to work or walking the dog. • Remember that even small amounts count; 10 minutes is better than none at all!
I don't like to exercise alone.	• Ask a family member, friend or neighbor to go walking with you. • Join a class. • Start up a walking group at work. • Walk at the local mall before the stores open.
I need a safe place to exercise.	• Invest in a piece of exercise equipment, such as a treadmill or stationary bike you can use at home. • Try using an exercise DVD. • Join a local walking club or sign up for a class. • Walk at the mall or the local park.
I'm afraid of low blood glucose and/or hurting myself.	• Check your glucose before you exercise and eat a small snack, if needed. • Bring a snack with you. • Choose activities that won't cause pain or injury. • Start slowly and stop if you get tired or feel pain. • Wear the right shoes and socks for physical activity.
I'm too tired to be active.	• You may feel tired at first but you'll soon have more energy. • Don't try to do too much, too soon. • Be active at a time of the day when you have the most energy.

Barriers	Suggestions
Exercise is boring.	• Choose something that you enjoy. • Try something new or different, such as a dance class or ice skating. • Distract yourself while you exercise: watch television or listen to music. • Exercise with someone.
I feel embarrassed.	• Try exercising at home until you feel more confident. • Sign up for a few lessons with a personal trainer. • Join a health club that offers programs geared towards what you need, such as a "women only" facility.
It's too expensive.	• Look into programs or classes at the local Y. • Ask someone to go walking with you. • Check into your healthcare coverage benefits; many offer a discount at certain health and fitness clubs. • Borrow exercise DVDs from the library.
I have neuropathy (pain in my legs and feet)	• Try a low-impact activity, such as swimming, water aerobics or using a rowing machine. • Consider renting or buying an "armchair exercise" DVD or ask an exercise physiologist or personal trainer to show you some exercises that can be done sitting in a chair.

Tips for Staying Active

For some people, starting a physical activity program is the easy part. But after a while, they become bored with their usual routine or find that they dislike what they're doing. Here are some ideas to help you stick with your activity plan:

- To prevent boredom, choose at least two different kinds of activity.

- Use a pedometer. Put it on in the morning and see how many steps you take in an average day, then try to increase that number each week until you reach your personal fitness goal. Aim for 10,000 steps each day.

- Try something new, such as ballroom dancing or a spinning class at the local Y.

- Join a walking or running club. Not only will you make new friends, they'll keep you going if you feel like giving up.

- Exercise with a family member, friend or neighbor. Keep track of your progress. Just as you record your blood glucose levels and food, recording the type and duration of activity can be helpful and will reinforce how hard you've been working.

- Enlist the support of your family and friends. Explain the role of activity in diabetes control. Make sure you set aside time in your day or evening to fit this in, and that your family understands that this is "your time."

- Start out gradually. Nothing can get you off track like sore muscles or having to gasp for breath.

- Think about the best time of day or night for you to exercise. Some people prefer to exercise first thing in the morning, while others prefer to be active after work. The best time to exercise is when it's best for you!

- Ask your healthcare team for help and support.

Exercising to Lose Weight

Exercise is an important part of any weight loss program, both to lose weight initially and to help keep the weight off once you've lost it. But even before you start to see any weight loss, eating less food and exercising can cause your blood glucose to improve very quickly–so quickly that you may not need as much diabetes medication as you once did. When you see your blood glucose going lower, call your healthcare provider for advice on using smaller doses of diabetes medication. And keep up the good work!

Try different types of activity to keep from getting bored.

Carry a Card

Carry a card that says you have diabetes. Put your name, address, phone number and your doctor's name and phone number on the card. Put the kind and amount of diabetes medication you take and the names of any other medicines you use on the card. Wear a bracelet or necklace with the same facts on it. Then people will be able to help you if you have a problem.

Carry Food

Always carry something with you to treat low blood glucose. Below are some suggestions.

Foods to Carry with You during Physical Activity
• 4 glucose tablets
• 1 tube of glucose gel
• 5 gummy or 8 regular Life Savers
• 2 tablespoons of raisins
• small juice box (4 ounces)

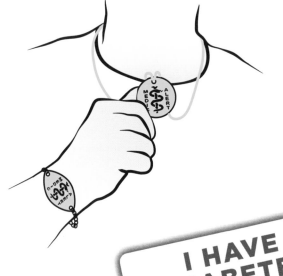

I HAVE DIABETES

I am not intoxicated. If I am unconcious or my behavior is peculiar, I may be having a reaction associated with diabetes or its treatment

I HAVE DIABETES
I may be having an insulin reaction. Please call a doctor or ambulance immediatly.
Name_____Phone No._____
Address _____
My Doctor is _____
Phone _____
My hospital is _____
My medication is _____

Chapter 4
Monitoring Your Blood Glucose

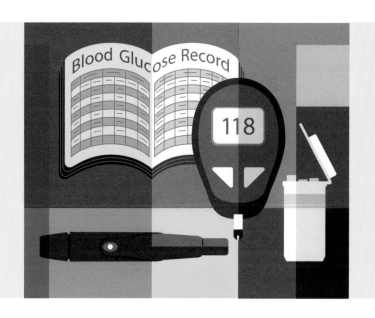

Why Monitoring Your Blood Glucose Is Important

Monitoring is an essential part of caring for your diabetes. There are two main ways to do this: 1) by having a hemoglobin A1C test at your healthcare provider's office, and 2) by checking your blood glucose at home using a blood glucose meter. It's important to remember that you can't tell how well your diabetes is doing by how you feel. You can feel fine even when your blood glucose levels are high. It is only by getting lab work done and checking blood glucose levels at home that you will know how well your diabetes is controlled.

What Is an A1C Test and What Does It Measure?

An A1C blood test: is the most important test to determine your overall diabetes control

The test:

- is an average of all your blood glucose results over the past two to three months
- is usually done two to four times each year
- measures the amount of glucose that attaches to hemoglobin, part of the red blood cells (the more glucose that attaches, the higher your A1C)

The A1C goal for most people with diabetes is less than 7%. Your goal may be different, however, so it's important to talk with your healthcare provider about the target that's best for you.

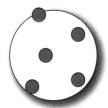

Non–diabetes range: 4–6%

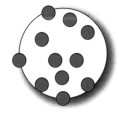

Goal A1C: less than 7%

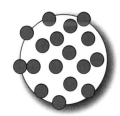

High A1C: 7% or higher

Why Is A1C Important?

Large studies have shown that keeping your A1C level under 7% will greatly reduce your risk for developing complications from diabetes, such as eye, kidney, nerve or heart problems.

What Do You Do if Your A1C Is above 7% or above Your Individual Target?

If your A1C is above your target, it tells you that your diabetes treatment plan needs a change. This could mean your meal plan needs adjustment, or you need a new medicine or your physical activity may need to be increased. Checking your blood glucose at home more often and setting up an appointment to discuss the results with your healthcare provider are important steps to take if your A1C is too high.

Blood Glucose Monitoring

Why Should You Check Your Blood Glucose?

The A1C tells you how your diabetes is doing over a 2- to 3-month period. Home blood glucose monitoring (or "checking") gives you information about your diabetes on a daily basis. You'll learn how well your diabetes care plan is working and whether your blood glucose is in your target range throughout the day. Reviewing daily blood glucose levels will help you and your healthcare team make any needed changes to your meal plan, physical activity and medicines.

How Do You Check Your Blood Glucose at Home?

You can check your blood glucose with a small device called a glucose meter. Your healthcare team will help you learn how to use your meter. There are many different kinds of meters on the market and they all work in a similar way. If you have health insurance, it is best to call your healthcare plan to find out what meter is preferred. The blood glucose meter strips and lancets are usually covered by health insurance and will be cheaper for you if you use a meter preferred by your insurance company.

Useful Tips for Using Your Meter

Today's blood glucose meters are fairly easy to use and give accurate results. If you've never used a meter before, it's helpful to have your diabetes educator show you how and to watch you check your own blood glucose just to make sure you're doing it correctly and that you get as accurate a result as possible.

How to Get a Good Blood Sample

- Wash your hands in warm water. You don't need to use alcohol wipes.

- Massage your hands.

- Choose which finger you'll use. It helps to use a different finger each time to avoid soreness.

- Keep your hand below your waist when using your lancet to "prick" your finger.

- Apply gentle pressure, but don't squeeze your finger.

Keeping your A1C less than 7% can lower your risk of complications.

Control Solution: What Is It and How Do You Use It?

- Control solution is the liquid you use to make sure that your test strips are working properly. Check the expiration date on the bottle; discard it if it's expired. Most control solutions are only good for three months once opened.

- Shake the control solution first, then use it like a drop of blood.

- Use control solution every couple of weeks, or sooner if you are questioning your blood glucose results.

- Control solution is not usually covered by insurance and can be purchased through your meter company or at a pharmacy.

Checking Your Blood Glucose: Important Reminders

- Make sure your strips are not expired. Check the date on the bottle.

- Make sure the code on your bottle matches the code on your machine.

- Make sure your hands are clean and dry.

- Do not use the center of your finger; it is the most sensitive area. Use a spot to the side of the center of your fingertip.

- Completely fill the strip target area with blood to make sure the results are accurate.

- You will need a prescription to have your glucose strips and lancets covered by insurance.

- There is usually an 800 number on the back of your meter for help with meter issues.

> Checking your blood glucose with a meter tells you how your diabetes is doing day to day.

How Often Do You Need to Check?

The type of diabetes medication you take or how high your A1C level is may determine when and how often you check your blood glucose. For example:

- If you take diabetes pills or take one injection of insulin each day, you will usually be asked to check twice a day, before breakfast and 2 hours after one meal, or as directed.

- If you take several insulin injections each day, you will usually be asked to check four times a day, before meals and at bedtime every day.

There will be times when you may need to check your blood glucose more often than usual. These include:

- during times of illness, surgery or stress

- when you are pregnant

- when you are starting a new diabetes medicine or changing your dose

- when you are taking a new medicine, such as steroids

- when other changes are made to your treatment program, such as changes to your meal plan or physical activity

- when you have higher or lower blood glucose readings than usual

What Should Your Blood Glucose Levels Be?

Your blood glucose level changes throughout the day. For example, it may be lower before you eat and higher after you eat. Discuss your target glucose range with your healthcare team.

Time of Check	Usual Target for Most People	Your Blood Glucose Targets
Before meals	70–130	
Two hours after meals	Less than 180	
Bedtime	90–150	

Your Blood Glucose Monitoring Action Plan:

Circle the days and times when you check:						
Days: Monday Tuesday Wednesday Thursday Friday Saturday Sunday						
Times: Before breakfast Before lunch Before dinner Bedtime						
After breakfast After lunch After dinner Middle of the night						

There are no "good" or "bad" glucose numbers!

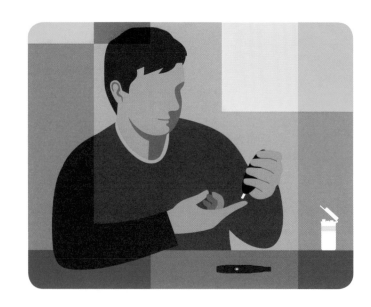

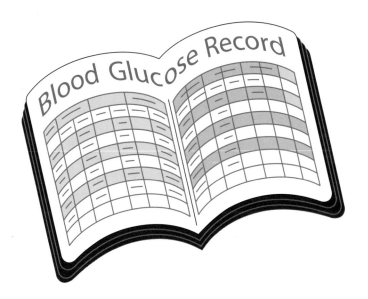

What to Do with the Results

Your blood glucose results are only helpful if you use them.

- *Write them down on a log sheet* or in a record book.

- *Look for patterns in your numbers.* All numbers are helpful; there are no "good" or "bad" numbers. It might help you to circle your lows in blue and your highs in red to better help you see patterns.

- *Take your results to your appointments.* They will help your healthcare team make better decisions about your diabetes treatment plan.

- *Call your healthcare provider* if the numbers are below 70 or above 250.

Alternate Site Checking

Most meters allow for what is called "alternate site testing." This means you can use sites other than the fingertips to get blood samples. These alternate sites include the upper arm, the forearm, the palm, the thigh and the calf. Check your meter instructions to see if you can use alternate site testing and which sites can be used. One benefit to alternate site checking is that it hurts less than using the fingertips to check. A disadvantage is that it can be hard to get enough blood and so the alternate site is sometimes not as accurate as the fingertip.

There are times when you shouldn't use an alternate site (see below). Patients who have blood glucose levels that change rapidly (such as in type 1 diabetes) should avoid alternate site checking.

Alternate site checking should NOT be used:

- if you think you are having a low blood glucose
- if you have recently exercised
- if you have eaten in the past three hours

What's New in Monitoring?

Estimated Average Blood Glucose (eAG)

When you get your lab results, you may see a number that appears along with your A1C called the "estimated Average Glucose" or eAG. An eAG is a new way to present an A1C value in numbers like those you see on your blood glucose meter. Understanding how eAG correlates with the A1C can help you better understand how your daily blood glucose readings relate to your long-term diabetes control.

Why use the eAG? Using eAG is simple because it's much like reading the numbers that you get from your blood glucose meter. Another reason to use eAG is that it may help you better understand how your day-to-day blood glucose readings relate to your longer-term diabetes control, and can help you and your healthcare team make any needed changes to your diabetes treatment plan.

The table below shows how your A1C level is expressed as eAG.

A1C Values Expressed as Estimated Blood Glucose Values		
A1C	Estimated Average BG	Estimated BG Range*
12	298	240-347
11	269	217-314
10	240	193-282
9	212	170-249
8	183	147-217
7	154	123-185
6	126	100-154
5	97	76-120

95% confidence interval

However, your blood glucose changes all the time, so it's helpful to know the range of your blood glucose readings, not just the eAG or A1C. The last column in the table, below left, tells you just that. So, for example, if your A1C is around 8%, in general, your average blood glucose is 183 mg/dl. The "95% confidence interval" means that 95% of the time your actual glucose averages (if you were checking your glucose thousands of time over three months) would be between 147 and 217.

Continuous Glucose Monitoring

Continuous glucose monitoring, or CGM, is a new technology that measures glucose readings every one to five minutes, 24 hours a day.

CGM is a system consisting of three components: a disposable sensor, a transmitter, and a receiver. The CGM system is used in addition to, not as a substitute for, checking your blood glucose with a meter. CGM is usually used by people who want to intensively manage their diabetes and are either using an insulin pump or taking several daily insulin injections. Patients who are started on CGM are usually followed regularly by an endocrinologist.

Chapter 5
Diabetes Pills

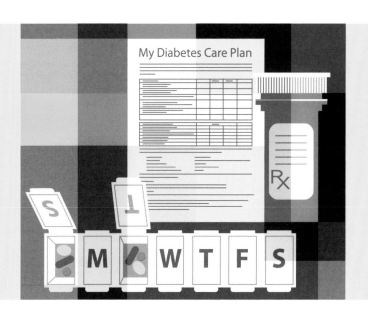

My Diabetes Care Plan

Facts about Diabetes Pills

Many different types of pills are available to treat type 2 diabetes. These pills can be used alone or in combination with one another and with insulin. Diabetes pills are one tool to help you manage your blood glucose in addition to following a meal plan and being physically active.

Based on new research and clinical trial results, new diabetes pills are approved almost every year. Ask your healthcare provider about new advances and treatment options that might help you.

What to Expect
Over Time Your Diabetes Will Change—and so Will Your Medicine.

Newly Diagnosed and Year One	Next Several Years	Longer than 10 years
One medicine along with watching carbohydrate intake and increasing physical activity is usually enough to control blood glucose levels.	Your A1C and blood glucose levels may start to go up. Additional diabetes medicine (pills, insulin, other injectables) may be needed.	A1C becomes harder to control with just pills. For many, insulin is needed in addition to pills.

How Diabetes Pills Work

With type 2 diabetes, you may have one or more of the following:

- a liver that releases too much glucose
- a pancreas that doesn't make enough insulin
- muscle cells that don't use insulin very well
- lower levels of gut hormones (hormones made in the small intestine)

Different types of diabetes pills address different problem areas, which is why a person with diabetes will often be on more than one kind of pill.

Your healthcare provider will help you determine which pill or pills will work best for you based on your blood glucose numbers.

- **Pills targeting the liver (biguanides):** Metformin and metformin extended release (brand names: Glucophage, Glucophage XR, Fortamet, Riomet, Glumetza) keep the liver from making too much glucose, especially overnight. Most people with type 2 diabetes start on metformin. It is even given to people who have prediabetes to help prevent blood glucose levels from rising.

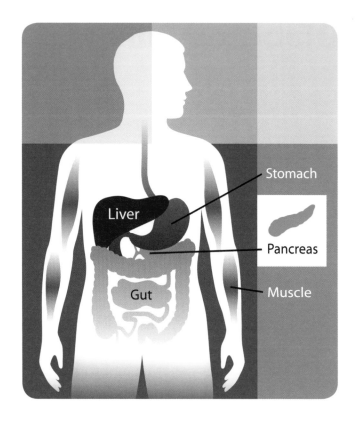

Over time you will need more medicine to control diabetes. This does not mean your diabetes is worsening; it just means your pancreas is making less insulin.

- **Pills targeting the pancreas (sulfonylureas and glinides):** These pills, such as glipizide, glyburide, glimepiride, repaglinide and nateglinide, help the body make more insulin, particularly at mealtime. If your blood glucose levels suddenly start to rise above 180 two hours after your meal, it may be a sign that you need this type of pill.

- **Pills targeting the muscle (thiazolidinediones or "TZDs"):** Currently Actos (pioglitazone) is the main TZD that's used. Actos increases the body's sensitivity to insulin, allowing insulin to help move glucose from the blood stream into the cell more easily. If your blood glucose levels are high all the time, your healthcare provider may recommend a TZD.

- **Pills targeting glucose absorption in the gut: (acarbose and miglitol):** These pills slow the movement of carbohydrate foods through the small intestine, allowing for glucose to be absorbed more slowly.

- **Pills targeting gut hormones (DPP-4 Inhibitors):** Sitagliptin, saxagliptin and linagliptin are part of a newer class of medicines called DPP-4 inhibitors. These medicines work by slowing the breakdown of gut hormones. These gut hormones, called GLP-1 hormones, help the body make more insulin at mealtime and slow the movement of food through the stomach. DPP-4 inhibitors also signal the pancreas to release more insulin while signaling the liver to release less glucose.

Important Tips about Taking Diabetes Pills

Here are some important tips to follow, no matter what diabetes pill(s) you take.

1. Take the dose that's prescribed by your healthcare provider.

2. Take it at the right time. Some pills are to be taken before the meal or with the first bite of the meal. See the Diabetes Pills Summary table at the end of this chapter.

3. If you miss a dose, write it down in your log book. DO NOT take an extra dose.

4. Do not change how many pills you take without asking your provider.

5. Check your blood glucose at the times specified by your provider or your diabetes team. If your blood glucose or A1C is within target most of the time, the dose is working. If not, check whether you have been eating the right amount and types of food or whether you have forgotten to take the right amount of medication. If your blood glucose remains high for a few weeks, contact your healthcare provider. A change in dose may be needed.

6. Do not take pills past their expiration date.

7. Diabetes pills are not approved for use during pregnancy. If you are pregnant or planning to become pregnant, talk to your healthcare provider about what to do. He or she most likely will take you off your diabetes pills and put you on insulin.

8. If you start a new medicine, let your provider know. Some other medicines can affect your diabetes. You may need a change in your diabetes pills.

Diabetes Pills Summary

Listed below are the various types of diabetes pills that are available and information on how to take them, how they work and their side effects.

Diabetes Pills	How to Take	How They Work	Side Effects	Of Note
Biguanides Metformin (Glucophage) Metformin liquid (Riomet) Metformin extended release (Glucophage XR, Fortamet, Glumetza)	**Metformin:** usually taken twice a day with breakfast and evening meal **Metformin extended release:** usually taken once a day in the morning	Decrease amount of glucose released from liver	Bloating, gas, diarrhea, upset stomach, loss of appetite (usually within the first few weeks of starting); take with food to minimize symptoms. Metformin is not likely to cause low blood glucose. In rare cases, lactic acidosis may occur in people with abnormal kidney or liver function.	Always tell your healthcare providers that you are taking these medicines as they may need to be stopped when you are having an imaging study using contrast dye or a surgical procedure.

Diabetes Pills	How to Take	How They Work	Side Effects	Of Note
Sulfonylureas Glimepiride (Amaryl) Glyburide (Diabeta, Micronase) Glipizide (Glucotrol, Glucotrol XL) Micronized glyburide (Glynase)	Take with a meal once or twice a day	Stimulate the pancreas to release more insulin, both right after a meal and then over several hours	Low blood glucose, occasional skin rash, irritability, upset stomach	Because these medicines can cause low blood glucose, always carry a source of carbohydrate with you. Follow your meal plan and activity program. Call your healthcare provider if your blood glucose levels are consistently low. If there is an increase in your activity level or reduction in your weight or calorie intake, the dose may need to be lowered.
Meglitinides Repaglinide (Prandin) **D-Phenylalanine Derivatives** Nateglinide (Starlix)	Both of these medications should be taken with meals. If you skip a meal, skip the dose.	Stimulate the pancreas to release more insulin right after a meal	Effects diminish quickly so pills must be taken with each meal; may cause low blood glucose	These work quickly when taken with meals to reduce high blood glucose levels. However, they are less likely than sulfonylureas to cause low blood glucose.

Diabetes Pills	How to Take	How They Work	Side Effects	Of Note
Thiazolidine-diones (TZDs) Pioglitazone (Actos)	Usually taken once a day; take at the same time each day	Make the body more sensitive to the effects of insulin	May cause side effects such as swelling (edema) or fluid retention. Do not cause low blood sugar when used alone. Increased risk of congestive heart failure in those at risk	Increase the amount of glucose taken up by muscle cells and keep the liver from overproducing glucose; may improve blood fat levels Talk with your healthcare provider if you have the following symptoms: nausea, vomiting, fatigue, loss of appetite, shortness of breath, severe edema or dark urine.
DPP-4 Inhibitors Sitagliptin (Januvia) Saxagliptin (Onglyza) Linagliptin (Tradjenta)	Take once a day at the same time each day	Improve insulin level after a meal and lower the amount of glucose made by your body	Stomach discomfort, diarrhea, sore throat, stuffy nose, upper respiratory infection Do not cause low blood glucose	Can be taken alone or with metformin, a sulfonylurea or Actos. Tell your healthcare provider if you have any side effects that bother you or that don't go away.

Diabetes Pills	How to Take	How They Work	Side Effects	Of Note
Alpha-Glucosidase Inhibitors Acarbose (Precose) Miglitol (Glyset)	Take with first bite of the meal; if not eating, do not take	Slow the absorption of carbohydrate into your bloodstream after eating	Gas, diarrhea, upset stomach, abdominal pain	Take with meal to limit the rise of blood glucose that can occur after meals. These do not cause low blood glucose. Side effects should go away after a few weeks. If not, call your healthcare provider.

Diabetes Pills	How to Take	How They Work	Side Effects	Of Note
Bile Acid Sequestrants Colesevelam (Welchol)	Take once or twice a day with a meal and liquid	Work with other diabetes medications to lower blood glucose	Constipation, nausea, diarrhea, gas, heartburn, headache (may interact with glyburide, levothyroxine and contraceptives)	Primary effect, when used either alone or with a statin, is to lower LDL cholesterol; has blood glucose-lowering effect when taken in combination with certain diabetes medications. Before taking this medication, tell your healthcare provider if you have high triglycerides (blood fats) or stomach problems. If you take thyroid medication or glyburide, take them 4 hours before taking Welchol. Tell your healthcare provider if you have side effects that bother you or that don't go away.

Diabetes Pills	How to Take	How They Work	Side Effects	Of Note
Combination Pills Pioglitazone & metformin) (Actoplus Met) Glyburide & metformin (Glucovance) Glipizide & metformin (Metaglip) Sitagliptin & metformin (Janumet) Sitagliptin & metformin ER (Janumet XR) Sitagliptin & simvastatin (Juvisync) Saxagliptin & metformin (Kombiglyze, XR) Linagliptin & metformin (Jentadueto) Repaglinide & metformin (Prandimet) Pioglitazone & glimepiride (Duetact)	Check with your provider; usually taken once a day	Combines the actions of each pill used in the combination	Side effects are the same as those of each pill used in the combination. Some combination pills may lead to low blood glucose levels if one of the medications contained in the combination has this effect. Some combination pills may contain a different type of medication, such as a statin. Ask your provider about possible side effects.	May decrease the number of pills you need to take.

Notes and Reminders

_____

_____

_____

_____

_____

_____

_____

_____

_____

_____

_____

_____

_____

Chapter 6
Insulin and Other Injectables

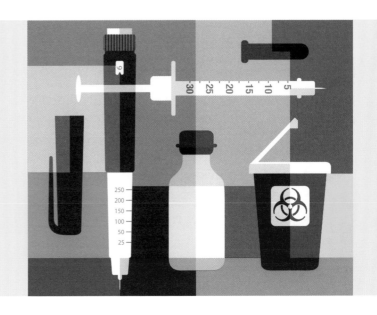

Insulin Facts

There are several things you should know about insulin.

- Insulin is a hormone that lowers blood glucose.

- Injected insulin replaces what the body makes naturally. People with type 1 diabetes must take insulin to survive.

- About half the people with type 2 diabetes will need to take insulin at some point in their lives. Taking insulin doesn't mean you've failed; your body may just need extra help.

- Insulin is safe and one of the most effective ways to lower blood glucose. It is measured in units just as milk is measured in pints and quarts.

- Insulin is made in different strengths. Most people use a strength called U-100.

- Insulins come in several different types. Some are faster-working and last for a shorter period of time while others are slower-working and last for a longer period of time.

- Different companies make different types of insulin. Always use the same brand and type of insulin that your provider has prescribed.

- Different injection sites (leg, stomach, etc.) may absorb some types of insulin at faster or slower rates. (See where to Inject Insulin later in this chapter.)

- The main side effect of insulin is that it can cause low blood glucose levels. Knowing how to recognize and treat lows is an important part of taking insulin (see Signs and Symptoms of Low Blood Glucose in Chapter 3).

Types of Insulin

All insulin is not the same. The types of insulin differ in:

- how fast they begin to work
- when they work their hardest
- how long they continue to work

There are two types and functions of insulin:

- **Background insulin (intermediate- and long-acting)**

  - Helps control glucose during the night and between meals

  - Take 1–2 times each day

  - **The Background insulins Are:**

    - ▲ NPH insulin: intermediate-acting and cloudy-looking

    - ▲ Glargine and detemir insulin: long-acting and clear-looking (also called "basal" insulins because they have no peak)

- **Mealtime insulin (rapid- and short-acting)**

  - Helps control glucose after eating a meal or a snack

  - Take before meals

  - You may need background insulin, mealtime insulin or both

- **The mealtime insulins are:**

  - ▲ Lispro, aspart and glulisine insulin: rapid-acting and clear-looking

  - ▲ Regular insulin: short-acting and clear-looking

- **Premixed Insulins**

  - Premixed insulins are a combination of background and mealtime insulin

  - Humulin 70/30 and Novolin 70/30 are premixed insulins that have some slower-acting (NPH) and some fast-acting (regular) insulin in one bottle

  - Humalog 75/25, Humalog 50/50 and NovoLog 70/30 also contain some slower-acting insulin along with some rapid-acting (lispro or aspart) insulin in one bottle

See the Usual Action Times table on the next page for the usual action times for the insulins described above.

Your provider will tell you:

- which brand of insulin to use
- what type or types of insulin to use
- how many units of each type to use
- what time(s) to inject insulin each day

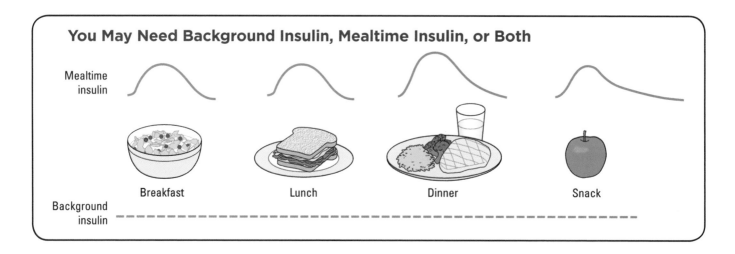

You May Need Background Insulin, Mealtime Insulin, or Both

Mealtime insulin

Breakfast   Lunch   Dinner   Snack

Background insulin

Usual Action Times

	Generic Name	Product	When to Take	When Starts	Works Best	How Long It Lasts
Mealtime Insulin						
Rapid-acting	aspart glulisine lispro	NovoLog Apidra Humalog	0–15 min before meal	10–30 min	30 min–3 hrs	3–5 hrs
Short-acting	Regular (R)	Humulin R Novolin R	30 min before meal	30–60 min	2–5 hrs	Up to 12 hrs
Background Insulin						
Intermediate-acting	NPH (N)	Humulin N Novolin N	Does not need to be given with a meal	90 min–4 hrs	4–12 hrs	Up to 24 hrs
Long-acting	detemir glargine	Levemir Lantus	Does not need to be given with a meal	45 min–4 hrs	Minimal Peak	Up to 24 hrs

Injecting Insulin

1. Insulin must be injected with a syringe or pen or delivered by an insulin pump. It cannot be taken by mouth.

2. For mealtime insulin, the usual injection time is 0–15 minutes before meals for lispro, aspart or glulisine and 30 minutes before meals for Regular insulin. However, if your blood glucose is high, you may want to wait a little longer to eat after injecting. For long- or intermediate-acting insulins (glargine, detemir, NPH), taking the insulin at the same time each day is recommended.

3. An injection that contains one kind of insulin is called a single dose. An injection of two insulins given in the same syringe at the same time is called a mixed dose.

4. Detemir (Levemir) and glargine (Lantus) are insulins that cannot be mixed with other insulins. When injecting these two insulins, choose an injection site that is 2 to 3 inches away from where mealtime insulin has been given.

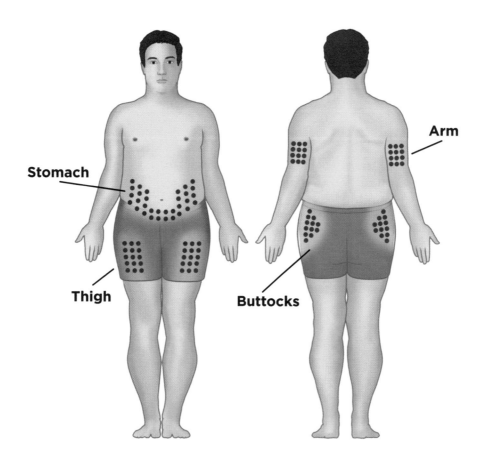

Stomach

Arm

Thigh

Buttocks

Where to Inject Insulin

You can inject insulin in four sites. Change your sites on a regular basis to avoid build up of scar tissue.

- Stomach: Inject at least two inches away from the navel, scars and moles.

- Arm: Inject into fatty tissue on the back of the upper arm between the shoulder and the elbow

- Thigh: Inject into the middle or outer part of thigh, at least 4 inches above the knee and at least 4 inches down from the top of the leg. The best area on the leg is the top and outer area of the thigh. Do not inject into the inner thigh.

- Buttocks: Inject into the hip or "wallet area."

It is important to change the sites where you inject insulin. If you use the same place over and over, the skin will get tough or lumpy and your insulin will not be absorbed properly.

For Regular insulin, the speed at which insulin is absorbed into your body differs depending on where you inject it. The abdomen absorbs most quickly, followed by the arm, the thigh and the buttocks. Ideally, it is best to choose at least two injection sites unless your provider tells you otherwise. Examples of how to rotate sites:

- Choose a site, such as the abdomen, and inject there for one month (rotating within the site). Then move to a new site.

- Choose a site for an injection time. For example, you may inject your morning insulin in your abdomen and your evening insulin in your thigh (rotate within the sites).

Insulin Syringes

Using an Insulin Syringe

There are several ways for you to inject insulin. One common way to inject is to use a syringe. Using a syringe means that you must "draw up" insulin from the vial into the syringe. Not all syringes are alike. If you decide to use a syringe, make sure you know the following:

- **Syringe size.** Insulin syringes come in three different sizes:
    - 3/10 cc syringe holds 30 units of insulin (one unit for each line on the syringe)
    - 1/2 cc syringe holds 50 units of insulin (one unit for each line on the syringe)
    - 1 cc syringe holds 100 units of insulin (two units for each line on the syringe)

One size syringe doesn't fit all. You should use the syringe size that best fits your insulin dose. For example, if you take 60 units of insulin, a ½ cc syringe that holds just 50 units wouldn't work too well because you'd need to give yourself another injection. In addition, ask your provider to prescribe the smallest size syringe that will work with your dose of insulin. Using the right syringe will help you be more accurate when drawing up your insulin.

- **Needle length.** There are two needle lengths available for syringes.
    - A 1/2-inch needle is the original needle size. This is the longest-size needle.
    - A 5/16-inch needle is a shorter needle and is more commonly used.

Because of the length of syringe needles, you must pinch up your skin before you inject to make sure that insulin is correctly injected. Pen needles are available in shorter lengths and they do not require you to pinch up when you inject.

- **Needle gauge.** The gauge of a needle refers to its thickness. The higher the gauge, the thinner the needle. A 30-gauge needle is thinner than a 28-gauge needle, for example. Syringe needles come in 32, 31, 30, 29 and 28 gauge.

Your provider or diabetes educator can help you choose the syringe size, needle length and needle gauge that's best for you.

> **One size syringe doesn't fit all. Use the syringe size that best fits your insulin dose.**

How to Draw Up Single and Mixed Doses of Insulin

It is important to learn how to draw up and inject insulin. There are two ways to do it. If you draw up a single dose (one type of insulin), use the first way. If you draw up a mixed dose (two types of insulin), use the second way.

Single Dose

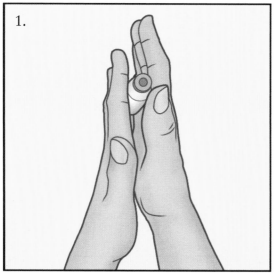

Roll the bottle if using cloudy insulin, until insulin is mixed. Skip this step for clear insulin.

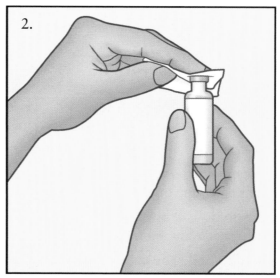

Wipe top of bottle with alcohol swab.

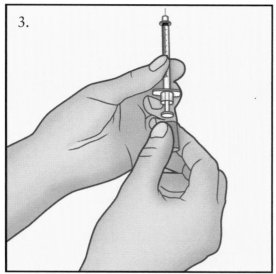

Take caps off of needle and plunger. Pull plunger down to _____ units.

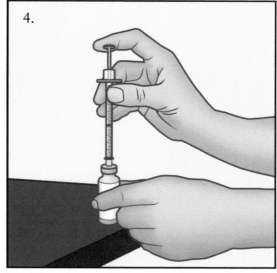

With bottle on table, put needle into bottle. Push plunger down to push air into bottle.

Single Dose (continued)

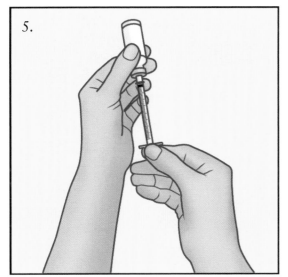

Turn bottle upside down.

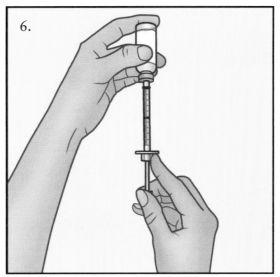

Pull plunger half way down to draw insulin into the syringe.

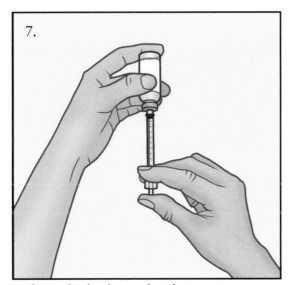

Push insulin back into bottle.

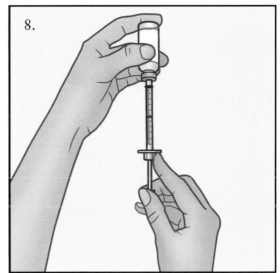

Pull plunger to _____units. Check for air bubbles. If air bubbles are present, push insulin back into bottle and repeat steps 7 & 8.

Mixed Dose

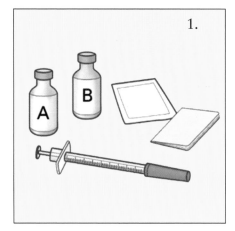

Gather insulin supplies.

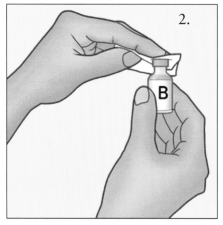

Roll NPH insulin (cloudy).
Wipe top of bottle with alcohol.

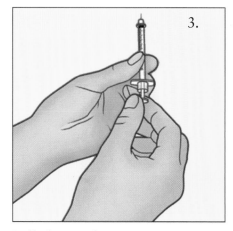

Pull plunger down to ___ units equal to NPH insulin dose.

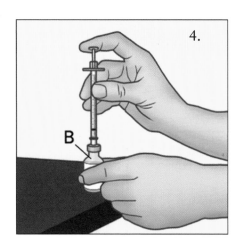

With bottle on table, put needle into bottle of NPH insulin and push air into bottle. Then remove needle.

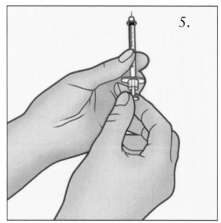

Pull plunger to ____units equal to clear insulin.

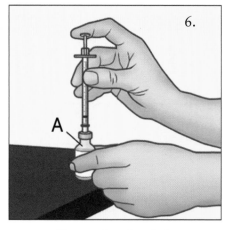

Put needle into bottle of clear insulin. Push air into bottle and leave needle in bottle.

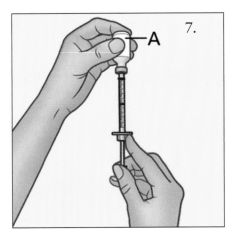

Turn bottle upside down. Pull plunger half way down the syringe. Then push insulin back into bottle.

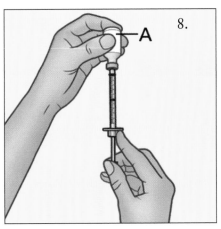

Pull plunger down to _____ units of clear. Check for air bubbles. If air bubbles are present, push insulin back into bottle and repeat step 7.

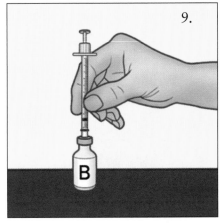

Put needle into NPH bottle and turn upside down.

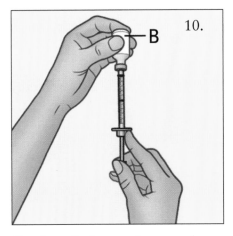

Slowly pull plunger down to the TOTAL dose. Total dose equal to _____ units (clear _____ + cloudy _____).

If you draw too much of the newly mixed insulin out, do not push insulin back into the bottle. Throw the syringe away and start over.

How to Inject Insulin with a syringe

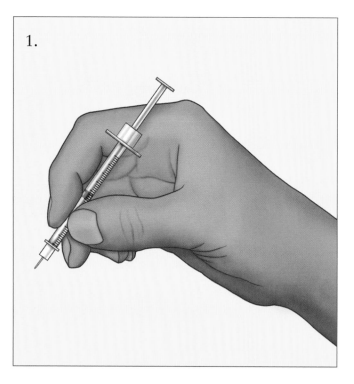

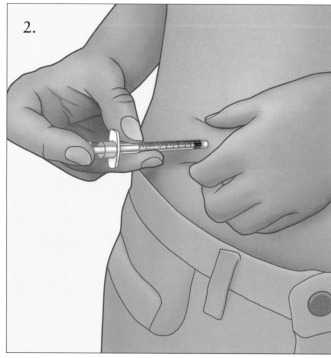

1. Hold the syringe like a pencil.

2. Pinch up the skin and inject. Push the needle straight into the skin at a 90 degree angle and push the plunger in.

3. Let go of the pinch and remove the needle. Dispose of the syringe in an appropriate container

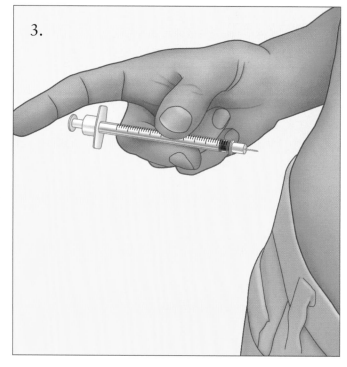

Insulin Pens

Using an Insulin Pen

Insulin pens are a convenient way to inject insulin. One of the main advantages of using an insulin pen is that it comes prefilled with insulin, doing away with the need to draw up the dose of insulin using a syringe and vial. This can be very helpful for people who have problems with their vision or for people who have difficulty holding a syringe and vial.

Pens are either disposable or reusable. Disposable pens come pre-filled with insulin and can be thrown away once the pen is empty or if the pen has been at room temperature for too many days. Reusable pens have a replaceable insulin cartridge that is thrown away after use. One type of pen is not better than the other. A benefit to reusable pens is that some of them allow you to dial-up half units of insulin, which is helpful if you take very small doses of insulin.

It's important to remember that you usually need a separate pen for each type of insulin that you take. For example, if you take both a mealtime and a bedtime (background) insulin, you will need two separate pens and will need to take two separate injections. The only exception to this is if you take a premixed insulin; then, only one pen is needed.

Pros and Cons of Using an Insulin Pen
Pros:

- Pens are easy, quick and convenient to use.
- Pens are helpful if you have difficulty seeing; you can listen for the "click" when dialing your dose. Each "click" is equal to one unit of insulin on most pens.

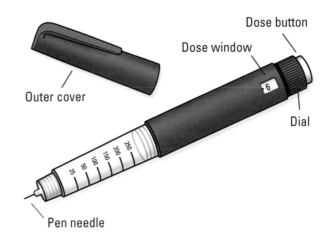

Outer cover — Dose window — Dose button — Dial — Pen needle

- Most pens hold 300 units of insulin whereas most insulin vials hold 1,000 units. If you take small doses of insulin, you'll waste less insulin using a pen than with a vial and syringe.

Cons:

- Pens may cost more than using syringes and insulin vials.
- You can't mix two different insulins with a pen; you must use two different pens if you take two different types of insulin.
- If you take large doses of insulin, you will go through insulin pens faster than if you use a vial and syringe.

An insulin pen uses a pen needle that is screwed onto the pen and is changed after every injection. On the next page, you will find useful instructions for how to use an insulin pen. Most insulins are available in pen form.

How to Dial Up and Use an Insulin Pen

1.

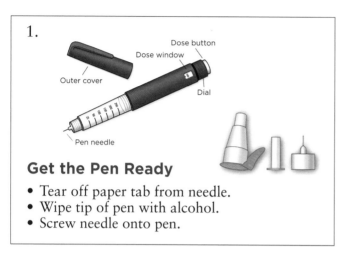

Get the Pen Ready

- Tear off paper tab from needle.
- Wipe tip of pen with alcohol.
- Screw needle onto pen.

2.

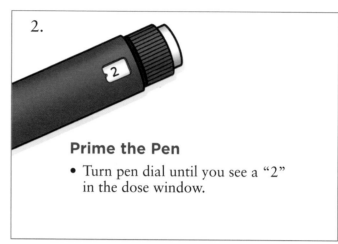

Prime the Pen

- Turn pen dial until you see a "2" in the dose window.

3.

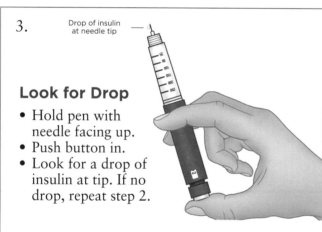

Look for Drop

- Hold pen with needle facing up.
- Push button in.
- Look for a drop of insulin at tip. If no drop, repeat step 2.

4.

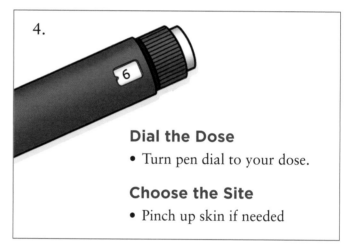

Dial the Dose

- Turn pen dial to your dose.

Choose the Site

- Pinch up skin if needed

5.

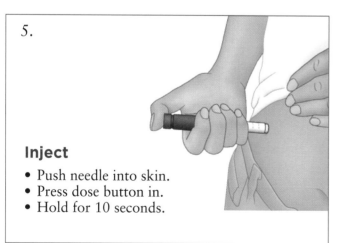

Inject

- Push needle into skin.
- Press dose button in.
- Hold for 10 seconds.

6.

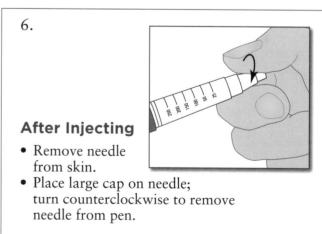

After Injecting

- Remove needle from skin.
- Place large cap on needle; turn counterclockwise to remove needle from pen.

Taking Care of Insulin, Syringes and Pen Needles

How Insulin in Bottles Should Be Stored

Store bottles of insulin that you are using at room temperature (59-86°) for about 1 month (28-30 days for most insulins; 42 days for detemir.). Do not keep bottles in a hot place like near a heater or in direct sunlight. Also, do not keep them near ice or in places where the insulin may freeze.

Do not use insulin after it has been kept at room temperature for longer than the manufacturer advises. Also, do not use insulin past the expiration date printed on the bottle, or if it looks different than usual. Unopened bottles of insulin and unopened insulin pens should be stored in the refrigerator and are good until the expiration date on the box and/or the bottle.

Look at your insulin daily and throw out the insulin if crystals or lumps are present.

How Insulin Pens Should Be Stored

Keep the pen that you are using at room temperature. It is good for:

- 42 days if detemir (Levemir)
- 28 days if lispro (Humalog), aspart (NovoLog) glulisine (Apidra) or glargine (Lantus)
- 2 weeks if NPH, 10 days if a mixed insulin, such as NovoLog 70/30, or Humalog 75/25
- Keep pens that you're not using in the refrigerator. Never freeze insulin pens or cartridges.

How to Dispose of Syringes and Insulin Pen Needles

Most people injecting insulin with syringes use plastic syringes which are made to be used once and then thrown away. It is not recommended that you re-use syringes. Pen needles should not be reused and should be changed after each use. Each city and town has its own rules for throwing away used needles. Check with local authorities about how to dispose of your "sharps". If your town doesn't have specific rules, check with a local hospital or local pharmacy. Always remember, safety is the best policy.

Step #1

- Use a strong plastic or metal container with a tight cap. All of your insulin syringes, pen needles and lancets should go into one of these containers after use. Do not throw sharps directly into the garbage.
- What's a good choice for a sharps container? Choose a container that is very strong so that the needles can't poke through the sides and with a lid that can be closed tightly to avoid spills.
  - A plastic bleach jug
  - A liquid detergent bottle
  - A plastic milk jug or other opaque or colored plastic bottle
- What is a poor choice for a sharps container?
  - A glass container (it can break)
  - A container that will be recycled or returned to a store (syringes, pen needles and lancets can't be recycled)
- DO NOT try to put the cap back on the needle or try to bend or break the needle.
- Keep the container in a place where small children or animals can't reach it.
- When the container gets full, put the lid or cap tightly onto your jug or bottle and seal it with tape.

Step #2

- When the container is full and tightly closed or sealed, make sure you know how to properly throw it away according to your local town or county regulations. Many towns and communities have needle disposal programs available. If you need additional information please go to the EPA's Website at www.epa.gov or www.safeneedledisposal.org/home.html.

Insulin Pumps

Insulin pumps are a more advanced tool for delivering insulin and are more commonly used by people who have type 1 diabetes. An insulin pump provides insulin 24 hours a day every day. The pump is loaded with insulin, which is then delivered by a plastic catheter that is inserted under the skin and left in place for 3 days at a time.

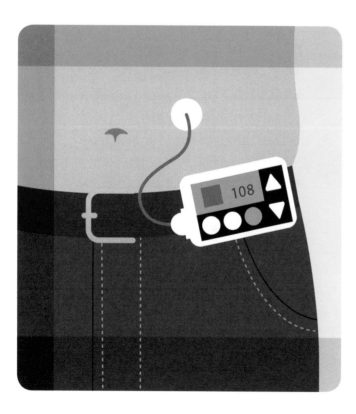

What Insulin Pumps Do:

- provide a level of background insulin 24 hours each day
- allow for adjustment in the amount of background insulin, depending on time of day and activity level
- allow for easy administration (called "bolusing") of insulin when eating

What Insulin Pumps Do NOT Do:

- measure your blood glucose level; that still requires using a glucose meter
- know what you are about to eat; only you know that
- automatically provide the right amount of insulin; you need to figure out the amount needed and tell the pump to administer it. While pumps can do math to assist in calculating the dose needed, the final decision is still made by the person wearing the pump.

Requirements for Using an Insulin Pump:

To use an insulin pump succesfully, you must:

- be willing to check blood glucose levels several times each day (at least 4)
- learn how to adjust insulin doses for various situations, such as high blood glucose, exercise and sick days
- understand pump mechanics and settings
- be able to assess the carbohydrate content of food (carb counting)
- be willing to wear the pump 24 hours each day, every day (except when you are showering, bathing, swimming or during intimate moments)

Other Injectable Diabetes Medicines

General Information

There are other diabetes medicines besides insulin that are injected. These medicines are synthetic forms of hormones that help control blood glucose.

For People with Type 2 Diabetes Who Do Not Take Insulin

Exenatide (Byetta)	Liraglutide (Victoza)
How it works	**How it works**
• Helps the body make the right amount of insulin at mealtime	• Helps the body make the right amount of insulin at mealtime
• Tells the liver to stop releasing glucose at mealtime	• Tells the liver to stop releasing glucose at mealtime
• Slows down digestion, helping to decrease hunger	• Slows down digestion, helping to decrease hunger
Facts to know about exenatide	**Facts to know about liraglutide**
• Can be taken alone or with certain types of diabetes pills	• Can be taken with certain types of diabetes pills
• Usually injected twice a day, 30-60 minutes before the morning and evening meals	• Injected once daily, at any time of day
• Does not typically cause low blood glucose (hypoglycemia); however, there is an increased risk for low blood glucose when it is taken along with a sulfonylurea, a type of diabetes pill	• Side effects include nausea and weight loss
	• Does not typically cause low blood glucose (hypoglycemia); however, there is an increased risk for low blood glucose when it is taken along with a sulfonylurea, a type of diabetes pill
• Side effects include nausea and weight loss	• Should not be used by people who have or are at risk for a rare form of thyroid cancer called medullary carcinoma or MTC
Injection technique: same technique and injection sites as used for insulin injections, except it should not be injected into the buttock area	**Injection technique:** same technique and same injection sites as used for insulin injections, except it should not be injected into the buttock area

Exenatide ER (Bydureon)

For People with Type 2 Diabetes <u>Who DO NOT Take Insulin</u>

How it works

- Works the same as exenatide. See exenatide section: 'How it works' for details.

Facts to know about exenatide ER

- Is a long-acting form of exenatide
- Injected with a syringe
- Is injected once every seven days (weekly), at any time of day, with or without meals
- Can be taken alone or with certain types of diabetes pills
- Does not typically cause low blood glucose (hypoglycemia); however, there is an increased risk for
- low blood glucose when it is taken along with a sulfonylurea, a type of diabetes pill.
- Side effects include nausea and weight loss

Pramlintide (Symlin)

For People with Type 2 Diabetes <u>Who Take Insulin</u>

How it works

- Slows down digestion, helping to decrease hunger
- Tells the liver to stop releasing glucose at mealtime

Facts to know about pramlintide

- Designed to be used by people who are already taking rapid-acting insulin with meals and long acting insulin.
- Injected up to four times daily with meals
- Low blood glucose may occur since it's taken at the same time as premeal insulin
- Side effects include nausea and weight loss

Injection technique: Injected the same way as insulin. Recommended sites are the thigh or abdomen. Close attention needs to be paid to rotation of sites with this drug; do not inject the rapid-acting insulin and pramlintide in the same area.

Chapter 7
Managing High or Low Blood Glucose

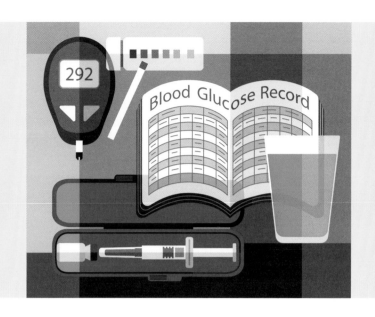

Why Managing Your Blood Glucose is Important

When you have diabetes, it is important to keep your blood glucose level from going too high or too low. High blood glucose levels, if left untreated, over time can cause complications. Low blood glucose levels if left untreated can cause a person to become confused and in rare cases to pass out or have a seizure. Knowing the causes of high and low blood glucose and how to recognize the symptoms and treat both conditions is an essential part of caring for your diabetes.

Remember: Most people with diabetes will have high and low blood glucose at some point, even if their diabetes is well controlled. The goal is to keep the highs and lows to a minimum and know how to treat them when they do occur.

High Blood Glucose (Hyperglycemia)

What Is High Blood Glucose?

High blood glucose is usually defined as a blood glucose over 140 mg/dl before a meal or over 180 mg/dl 2 hours after a meal. If your blood glucose levels are consistently above these

targets an adjustment to your treatment plan may be needed. If you are an older adult (over 70), have problems recognizing low blood glucose levels or have other serious health problems, your glucose goals may be higher. Ask your healthcare provider what your target goals are.

What Are the Symptoms of High Blood Glucose?

The most common symptoms of high blood glucose are:

- increased thirst
- increased urination
- dry mouth or skin
- tiredness or fatigue
- increased hunger
- blurred vision
- more frequent skin or vaginal infections
- slow-healing cuts and sores
- unexplained weight loss

However, you may not have any symptoms and still have high blood glucose levels. This is why checking your blood glucose with your meter is so important.

Are you at risk for high blood glucose? Below, on the left, are listed some typical causes of high blood glucose. On the right are some explanations for the causes. Are there any changes you could make to lower your glucose numbers? Check any that apply to you.

Causes of High Blood Glucose	Explanations for the Causes
Too much food	☐ You sometimes eat more food than usual. ☐ You've changed your eating schedule. ☐ You've changed the types of foods that you've been eating. ☐ You've been eating high-fat foods.
Not enough physical activity	☐ You've been doing less physical activity lately. ☐ You are not doing enough/any physical activity.
Taking diabetes medication at the wrong time	☐ You haven't been taking your diabetes medication at the right time.
"Bad" or spoiled insulin	☐ Your insulin looks different (cloudy, clumpy) than it usually does. ☐ Your insulin has been exposed to very hot or very cold temperatures. ☐ Your insulin has expired.

How to Take Care of High Blood Glucose

1. Drink plenty of water or sugar-free beverages so that you don't become dehydrated. Aim for at least 8 glasses each day.

2. For several days, check your blood glucose more often: before meals, at bedtime and occasionally 2 hours after the meal. Write down the numbers in your log book.

3. Look for a pattern. For example, do most of your high glucose readings occur after dinner?

4. Try to determine the cause. Perhaps you've been eating more than usual or forgetting to take your diabetes medicine.

5. Make a plan to correct it.

6. If you are unsure of what to do, make an appointment with your healthcare provider.

> **Diabetes changes over time. You may need more medicine, including insulin.**

Your healthcare provider may recommend that you change or increase your diabetes medicine if your high blood glucose can't be explained by food or physical activity. Don't change your diabetes medicine without first talking with your healthcare provider or at least having instructions from him or her on how to do so on your own.

The need for more diabetes medicine over time is a normal, expected change in the treatment of your diabetes and is a result of the natural progression of type 2 diabetes. Over time, the insulin-producing cells in your pancreas are unable to make enough insulin, which means that more or different types of medicine, including insulin, are needed to keep you healthy.

Taking Care of High Blood Glucose When You Are Sick

A cold, upset stomach, flu, infection, or any illness or injury may cause high blood glucose. Follow the sick-day rules in Chapter 8 if you are ill.

Unexplained High Blood Glucose

Sometimes your blood glucose may become high even when you are feeling well and taking good care of your diabetes. If you have type 1 diabetes and your blood glucose is over 250 and you don't know why, it is important to check your urine for ketones.

Checking Your Urine for Ketones

What Are Ketones?

Ketones are acid substances made when your body does not have enough insulin and starts to burn fat for energy. This can occur with severe calorie restriction, such as with very low carb diets, when a person is vomiting or when a person with diabetes does not have enough insulin.

There are three significant times when the body may not have enough insulin and ketones may start to become a problem:

1. when you are first diagnosed with type 1 diabetes

2. when you have type 1 diabetes and are not taking insulin as prescribed

3. when you are ill and have type 1 diabetes, or when you are ill, have type 2 diabetes and take multiple daily injections of insulin

Ketones are much less common in people with type 2 diabetes than type 1 diabetes.

Without enough insulin, glucose starts to build up in the bloodstream and the body breaks down fat, instead of glucose for energy. When fat is broken down, ketones form. As ketones start to build up in the bloodstream, they spill into the urine. If ketone levels are allowed to go too high, they can make the blood acidic and cause an emergency situation called diabetes ketoacidosis. This is why it's important for people with type 1 diabetes to know when and how to check for ketones.

How to Check for Ketones

You can check to see if your body is making ketones by doing a simple urine test or by using a special meter to check the blood for ketones. Ketone strips for testing urine can be purchased, without a prescription.

To test your urine for ketones, follow the steps below:

1. Dip a ketone test strip in a cup of urine.

2. Carefully follow the directions that come with the strips. Correct timing is very important. Wait for the strip to change color.

3. The color it changes to depends on the level of ketones in the urine. Match the color with the colors on the test strip instructions. The test result can be negative, or show small, moderate or large numbers of ketones.

When to Check for Ketones

If you have type 1 diabetes or have type 2 diabetes and are on multiple daily injections of insulin:

- Check your urine for ketones when your blood glucose is over 250 for two tests in a row and you do not know why, or when you are planning to exercise and your blood glucose is over 250.

- It is very important to check for ketones when you are ill and your blood glucose is over 250. Often illness, infections or injuries will cause sudden high blood glucose levels.

What should you do if the ketone test is positive?

- Call your doctor or other healthcare provider; you may need additional rapid-acting insulin.

- Drink plenty of water and sugar-free fluids to "wash out" the ketones.

- Continue checking your blood glucose every 3–4 hours; check for ketones if the blood glucose is over 250.

- Do not exercise if your blood glucose is over 250 and ketones are present.

If ketones are present, follow your sick-day plan. If you are unsure of what to do on a sick day, see the sick-day rules in Chapter 8 and call your healthcare provider. If you have type 1 diabetes, high blood glucose levels if left untreated can lead to a serious condition called DKA (diabetic ketoacidosis)

DKA (Diabetic Ketoacidosis)

DKA is a serious medical condition that affects people with type 1 diabetes, but sometimes affects people with type 2 diabetes who take insulin, as well. If you are ill, have not been taking your insulin, or if your insulin pump is not working correctly, you are at risk for DKA. With DKA, your body cannot use sugar (glucose) for energy, and breaks down fat instead. When fat is used for energy, an acid substance called ketones forms in the blood and flows into your urine. Blood glucose levels of 250 or higher for several days or weeks can be a warning sign of DKA, although DKA can occur very quickly when you're sick or if your insulin pump isn't working correctly. The combination of high blood glucose and ketones can lead to DKA if not treated quickly.

> **If you have DKA, you must be taken to a hospital.**

You may get DKA quickly if you are sick. To prevent DKA when you are ill or have an infection, check your blood glucose every 4 hours and if it's 250 or higher, check your urine for ketones. Follow your sick-day plan. If you do not have a sick-day plan and ketones are present, call your provider right away. You may need to go to the hospital for treatment. (See Chapter 8 on Sick-Days Rules.)

Symptoms of DKA

Be alert for signs and symptoms of DKA, especially when you are sick. Symptoms include:

- having to urinate a lot
- being very thirsty or hungry
- feeling sleepy
- feeling weak
- vomiting
- stomach pains
- chest pains
- rapid breathing

Having any of these symptoms doesn't mean that you have DKA, but you should call your healthcare provider if they do occur. If you have DKA, you must be taken to a hospital for treatment.

When to Call Your Healthcare Provider

Call your healthcare provider if your blood glucose is 250 or higher for more than 2 readings AND you:

- feel ill
- have a fever
- feel sick to your stomach (nausea)
- are vomiting
- are having or have recently had surgery
- are unsure what to do

Low Blood Glucose (Hypoglycemia)

You can get low blood glucose levels if you are on certain diabetes pills or insulin. Low blood glucose is sometimes called "hypoglycemia" or "insulin reaction" and is very treatable. You may feel hungry, shaky, nervous, dizzy, weak or irritable. If your blood glucose level gets too low, you can get confused, fall, have an accident and in some rare cases, even pass out or have a seizure. That's why it's important to know how to recognize and treat low blood glucose.

What Is Low Blood Glucose?

Low blood glucose is a blood glucose below 70 mg/dl. It is a side effect of certain diabetes medications. Signs and symptoms of lows can occur when your blood glucose falls below 70 mg/dl or when your blood glucose drops quickly even though levels are in the normal range.

What Are the Warning Signs of Low Blood Glucose?

You may feel:	You may have:	To others you may appear to:
dizzy	a headache	have an unsteady walk
shaky	difficulty concentrating	have trouble focusing
sweaty	confusion	be irritable before meals
irritable	blurred vision	be acting differently
weak	increased hunger	
	no symptoms	

Hypoglycemia Unawareness

Some people who have had diabetes for many years have difficulty knowing if they are "low" because they no longer have the usual symptoms of low blood glucose. This is a condition called "hypoglycemia unawareness". If you have this condition, it means that your blood glucose has to drop even lower before you feel symptoms and this may cause you to delay treatment. If you think you may have hypoglycemia unawareness, work with your healthcare team to design a treatment program that will prevent low blood glucose as much as possible. You may also need to increase your target glucose goals to keep you safe.

"Hypoglycemia unawareness" is the name given to the condition of not feeling the usual symptoms of low blood glucose.

What Causes Low Blood Glucose?

Causes of Lows	Are you at risk for low blood glucose? Check any below that apply to you
Too little food	☐ You sometimes skip or delay your meal or snack. ☐ You drink alcohol without eating. ☐ You eat different amounts of carbohydrate from meal to meal.
Not planning for physical activity	☐ You do not check your blood glucose before physical activity. ☐ You do not know when to snack before physical activity. ☐ You sometimes exercise longer or harder than usual without snacking or checking your blood glucose. ☐ You do not adjust your insulin when you are physically active.
Too much medication	☐ You sometimes take your insulin and/or diabetes pills at the wrong time. ☐ You sometimes take extra diabetes pills or insulin.
Combination of these factors	☐ Yes ☐ No

Preventing Low Blood Glucose

You can reduce the chances of having low blood glucose by doing the following:

- Eat your meals at about the same times each day as much as possible.
- Don't skip meals.
- Don't drink alcohol on an empty stomach.
- Learn how to adjust your food and/or diabetes medicine for physical activity.
- Check your blood glucose as recommended by your healthcare team.
- Check your blood glucose if you think you may have a low blood glucose.

Important reminders:

- Always carry a "hypoglycemia treatment" with you (see list under 3. below).

- Wear identification stating that you have diabetes.

- Teach family, friends and coworkers to recognize the signs, symptoms and treatments of low blood glucose. If you take insulin, get an emergency glucagon kit.

- Monitor your blood glucose before and after physical activity. If low blood glucose levels are a problem, ask for help to balance your diabetes plan with your fitness program.

- Check your blood glucose before you drive or use heavy machinery, and every 60 to 90 minutes thereafter.

Steps for Treating a Low Blood Glucose

1. Check your blood glucose to confirm that it is low. You can't always go by how you are feeling. If your blood glucose falls below 70, or is at the low end of your target range, treat it immediately! If you are unable to check your blood glucose but think you are low, treat it anyway.

2. Stop what you are doing and sit down.

3. Take 15 grams of carbohydrate (carb) in the form of one of these hypoglycemia treatments:

   - 4 oz. (½ cup) regular fruit juice
   - 6 oz. regular soda (NOT diet)
   - 4 glucose tablets
   - 1 tube glucose gel
   - 1 Tbsp. sugar, honey or jelly
   - 8 oz. skim milk
   - 7 gummy or 8 regular Life Savers
   - 2 Tbsp. raisins (small box)

> **IMPORTANT!**
>
> **Don't treat hypoglycemia with chocolate, peanut butter or other high-fat foods. These foods are not absorbed quickly enough to raise your blood glucose.**

4. Recheck blood glucose after 10–15 minutes. If it is less than 80 mg/dl, repeat the treatment (step 3).

5. Follow your treatment with a meal or snack. This snack should contain 15 grams of carb. If your meal is more than an hour away, make sure to have 30 grams of carbohydrate.

6. Think about why the low blood glucose might have occurred. If you don't know why you went low, call your healthcare provider. You might need a change in your diabetes medication dose.

Insulin users who become unconscious or who are unable to swallow should not be given anything by mouth, due to the risk of choking.

> **Always carry carbohydrate with you if you're at risk for low blood glucose.**

When to Call Your Healthcare Provider

Call your healthcare provider if you have a low blood glucose and do not know what caused it, or if you needed the help of someone else to treat your low blood glucose. Your diabetes treatment plan may need to be changed.

What Is Glucagon?

Glucagon is a hormone, like insulin, that raises blood glucose. It's given as an injection when a person has a low blood glucose and cannot swallow, or is unconscious.

Do You Need Glucagon?

You should learn to use glucagon if you:

- have type 1 diabetes
- have ever lost consciousness from a low blood glucose
- take 3 or more injections of insulin a day or are on an insulin pump
- are unable to feel the symptoms of low blood glucose (hypoglycemic unawareness)

A glucagon emergency injection can be given by a friend, family member or co-worker if you are low and either can't swallow or pass out. You or your diabetes educator should spend time showing your family and friends how to use glucagon before you need it. If you take multiple injections of insulin each day or have passed out from lows in the past, talk to your healthcare provider about getting a glucagon kit. Glucagon is available by prescription at drug stores.

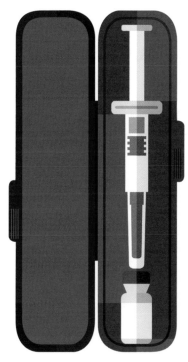

Glucagon Kit.

> **Make sure that family and friends know what to do if you lose consciousness or have other severe symptoms of a low blood glucose.**

Notes and Reminders

_____

_____

_____

_____

_____

_____

_____

_____

_____

_____

_____

_____

_____

_____

Chapter 8
Sick-Day Rules

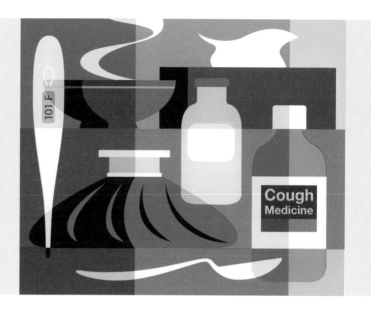

What Are Sick-Day Rules?

When you have diabetes, you need to take particularly good care of yourself when you're sick. Any illness, such as the common cold, the flu or a stomach bug, may cause high blood glucose. High blood glucose can also occur from an injury, surgery or certain dental procedures like having a tooth pulled. Emotional stress can raise blood glucose, too. When you're under any kind of stress, your body makes hormones that cause blood glucose levels to rise.

On days when you are sick, your blood glucose level can go high even when you are eating less. High blood glucose levels left untreated can lead to more serious medical problems, so it is important to have a plan. Below are the steps (called sick-day rules) you will want to follow when you are sick or recovering from surgery.

Sick-Day Rules

1. Always take your diabetes medication unless your healthcare provider tells you not to.

2. Check your blood glucose 4 times a day for mild illness and every 3–4 hours for more severe illness. It is important that you check your blood glucose often when you are ill because it can get high quickly and you will not be able to tell how high it is by how you are feeling. If you are too sick to check, ask someone to do it for you. If you take insulin, also check for ketones (see the section about checking your urine for ketones in Chapter 7) if your blood glucose is 250 or higher.

3. Call your healthcare provider if your blood glucose is 250 or higher for two blood glucose results. Do this whether you have ketones or not.

> **Never skip your pills or insulin even if you are too sick to eat.**

4. If you use insulin, you may need to take extra injections of insulin if your blood glucose is 250 or higher. You can learn how to adjust your insulin dose yourself or you can call your healthcare provider for help when you get sick. Either way, make sure that you have the right information or know whom to call if this happens.

5. Try to follow your meal plan as best you can when you're sick. It's important to eat and drink during this time. If you can't follow your meal plan but can still eat some food, choose items from the list on the next page. Each item on the list counts as one carbohydrate choice or 15 grams of carbohydrate.

6. If you feel too sick to eat, drink 6–8 ounces of liquids every hour. If you are unable to eat solid foods, you should switch back and forth between drinks that have sugar in them, such as regular soft drinks and juice, one hour, and drinks that do not contain sugar, such as diet soft drinks and tea or water, for the other hour. If you are unable to follow your meal plan, drink liquids that contain salt, such as clear soup, bouillon, tomato juice or Gatorade.

7. Rest and keep warm. Do not exercise. Have someone take care of you.

Treat the Underlying Illness

It's important that you treat the illness that has made you sick. Follow the directions from the provider who is caring for your illness. Take medications, such as antibiotics or over-the-counter pain relievers, as prescribed. Be sure to tell the provider who is caring for your illness that you have diabetes.

> Stay healthy: Get your flu shot every year. Ask for the pneumonia vaccine if you haven't already had one.

Over-the-Counter Medications

People with diabetes are often concerned about using over-the-counter medications, such as cough syrup, when they're sick. Sometimes sugar-free medications may not be available, but the amount of sugar in most medications is very small and is unlikely to raise your blood glucose. So, if sugar-free medications are available, they're fine to use, but you can also use the "regular" versions, too. Your pharmacist can answer any questions that you have about medications.

When to Call Your Healthcare Provider

Having a sick-day plan can make it easier to take care of your diabetes when you're not feeling well. But there may be times when you feel very sick or just aren't sure what to do. It's always best to be on the safe side and call your healthcare provider, especially if you:

- have constant nausea or diarrhea
- are vomiting or unable to keep fluids down
- have blood glucose levels over 250 for more than two readings
- are having low blood glucose levels
- have a fever lasting more than 24 hours
- have abdominal pain
- are unsure what to do

Sick-Day Foods

Good nutrition is important when you're sick. As best you can, follow your meal plan. Try to eat or drink the amount of carbohydrate that you usually take-in at your meals and snacks. If you don't have specific carbohydrate goals for your meals, think about meeting with a dietitian and, in the meantime, aim to consume at least 45 grams of carbohydrate every 3 to 4 hours. Lowfat, bland foods such as toast, crackers, soup, mashed potatoes, rice, pudding and yogurt are good choices. If you're not feeling sick to your stomach, also try to eat some lower-fat protein foods, such as eggs, lowfat cottage cheese or chicken breast.

The foods and beverages listed below each contain 15 grams of carbohydrate (one carb choice). Use these when you are ill and unable to follow your usual meal plan.

Applesauce	½ cup
Apple juice	½ cup
Grape juice	⅓ cup
Orange juice	½ cup
Fruited yogurt	⅓ cup
Milkshake	¼ cup
Eggnog	½ cup
Gatorade	1 cup
Honey	1 Tbsp.
Regular gelatin	½ cup
Regular pudding	¼ cup
Regular ice cream	½ cup
Sherbet	¼ cup
Twin-pop popsicle	1 pop
Hot cereal	½ cup

Other food choices that you may try include salty foods like broth, bouillon or tomato juice or soft solids like toast, hot cereals or soups.

A Sick-Day Checklist

Keep these items on hand in case you become sick:

☐ Sugar-free and regular gelatin (such as Jell-O) or popsicles

☐ Broth packets (salt-free if you are on a low-sodium diet)

☐ Saltine crackers (unsalted if you are on a low-sodium diet)

☐ Caffeine-free tea

☐ Caffeine-free carbonated beverages (sugar-free and regular)

☐ Substitute foods: fruit juice, applesauce, sherbet

☐ Thermometer

☐ Extra bottles of rapid-acting insulin and syringes, or insulin pens

☐ Medications to relieve fever, such as acetaminophen

☐ Antidiarrheal medications (Lomotil, Kaopectate, Pepto-Bismol)

☐ Telephone number of your diabetes care team

☐ Cold/cough/flu medicine recommend by your healthcare provider

☐ Ketone strips (if needed) for urine or blood.

☐ Glucagon kit (if taking insulin) in case of severe low blood glucose

Chapter 9
Foot Care

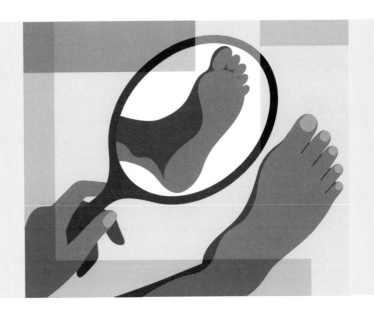

How Diabetes May Cause Foot Problems

Having diabetes puts you at risk for foot problems. Here's how:

- Diabetes can cause nerve damage in your feet. If this happens, you may not feel pain if, for example, you step on a tack. You might also not feel heat or cold.

- Diabetes may narrow your blood vessels. These narrowed blood vessels may not carry enough blood to your legs and feet, which may cause your legs to hurt when you walk. Cuts and scratches may heal slowly. Your feet may get red when walking or white when propped up on a chair.

- Having high blood glucose for a long time can put you at risk for infections that can be slow to heal.

- If you have difficulty seeing your feet or reaching down to check your feet, you may miss cuts, sores or signs of infection.

You can lower your chances of having foot problems by taking good care of your feet.

Daily Foot Care

1. Every day, look at your feet for dry skin, cracks, cuts or redness. Be sure to check the bottoms of your feet. If you can't bend over to see your feet, place a hand mirror on the floor and hold each foot over it. If you have trouble seeing, ask someone to check your feet for you. Call your healthcare provider if you find cuts or sores that don't seem to be healing. Redness, swelling and increased warmth are signs of infection.

2. Wash your feet in warm, soapy water every day. Don't soak your feet; soaking softens the skin and increases your risk for infection. Never use hot water, especially if you have nerve damage in your feet. Use gentle soap. Rinse your feet well and dry them carefully, especially between the toes.

3. After you've washed your feet, put lotion on them to keep the skin from getting dry. Do not put lotion between your toes. If your feet are very dry, apply the lotion at bedtime and put on clean, dry socks. Put talcum powder on your feet if they sweat. Dust off any extra powder.

4. File your toenails with an emery board. Never use scissors or clippers because you might cut yourself and get an infection. File your nails to follow the shape of your toes. Round the edges. Don't file them shorter than the ends of your toes. Ask someone to help you if you do not see well, or have a foot doctor (podiatrist) trim your toenails.

5. See a podiatrist if you have corns, calluses, ingrown toenails or fungal nail infections. Never perform "bathroom surgery" on your feet.

6. See a podiatrist regularly if you have poor circulation, nerve damage or thick toenails.

Choose unscented moisturizers that do not contain alcohol. Petroleum jelly and lanolin are good choices.

Shoes and Socks

Choosing the right footwear for your feet can help them stay healthy.

- **Wear good shoes.** Buy shoes that protect and cover your feet and that fit you well. When you buy shoes, shop in the afternoon when your feet are slightly swollen, and wear the socks or stockings that you plan to use with them. You may need specially made shoes if you have crooked toes or foot deformities. Check the insides of your shoes for pebbles or other objects before you put them on. Break in new shoes gradually to prevent blisters.

- **Don't go barefoot.** Always wear shoes, sandals or flip-flops, even when you're on the beach. Wear sturdy slippers when you're at home. Wear swimming shoes when you're on the beach or swimming in a pool or lake.

- **Wear the rights socks and stockings.** Wear socks made of material that wicks moisture away from the skin. Wear a clean pair of socks every day, and change your socks if your feet sweat a lot. Choose socks that are free of seams and darns. Don't wear socks or stockings that are too tight at the top.

Preventing Problems

Daily foot care and wearing the right shoes and socks can prevent foot problems. Here are some other suggestions:

- **Get a foot exam.** Make sure your healthcare provider does a foot exam at least once a year. You may need foot exams more often if you have neuropathy, poor circulation or a history of foot infections. Take off your shoes and socks when you're in the exam room to remind your provider to check your feet.

- **Protect your feet** from very hot or very cold temperatures. Avoid hot baths, heating pads, electric blankets, hot pavement and hot sand; if you have nerve damage, you might not be able to feel the heat.
- **Quit smoking.** Smoking decreases the amount of blood flowing to the foot.
- **Take care of cuts and scratches** right away.

First Aid

Take care of cuts and scratches right away.

- Wash them with warm water and soap. Do not soak.
- Use a gentle medicine such as ST 37, Bacitracin, or Neosporin.
- Cover with gauze and paper tape.
    - Do not use adhesive tape on your skin.
    - Avoid using plastic bandages.
- Check the cut or scratch two times a day.
- Stay off your feet as much as possible.

Call your doctor or healthcare provider if:

- cuts or scratches do not heal within 48 hours
- you notice any drainage
- you are unsure what to do

> **Take off your shoes and socks when in the exam room to remind your healthcare provider to check your feet.**

Notes and Reminders

WHAT YOU NEED TO KNOW ABOUT DIABETES

Chapter 10
Know Your Numbers and Lower Your Risk for Complications

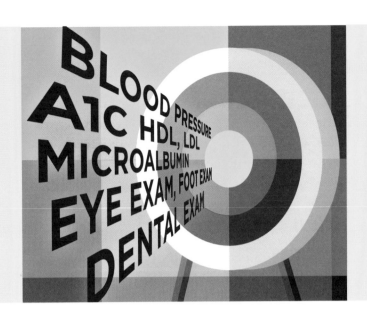

Why It Is Important to Know Your Numbers

There is a lot you and your healthcare team can do to reduce your risks for getting the complications of diabetes. The most common complications involve the heart, blood vessels, feet, eyes, kidneys and nerves. Keeping blood glucose levels in target range is only a first step. Controlling blood pressure and cholesterol is also important. In this chapter, you will learn about each of the ways for staying healthy. Be sure you have the described tests as often as recommended, and ask about your results.

> Large studies have shown that keeping your A1C level under 7% will greatly reduce your risk for developing complications from diabetes such as eye, kidney, nerve or heart problems.

The A1C Test

Much like you use a map or a GPS to help you find your way, your diabetes "numbers" can help you find your way when it comes to lowering your risk for diabetes complications. The A1C test is a gauge that lets you and your healthcare provider know how well your diabetes treatment plan is working.

The A1C reflects your average blood glucose readings over the past two to three months. How does this work? Glucose sticks to red blood cells as they travel throughout the body. Red blood cells live for about three months, so we can measure how much glucose sticks to them before they die.

Why the A1C Test Is Important

The A1C test is the single most important test for people with diabetes. Major studies, such as the Diabetes Control and Complications Trial (DCCT) and the United Kingdom Prospective Diabetes Study (UKPDS), show that high blood glucose over a long period of time will cause a lot of problems, or complications, including damage to your eyes, kidneys, and nerves. While not everyone with a high A1C will experience complications, since we don't know who will and who won't, the best advice is for everyone with diabetes to aim for their A1C target.

How It's Measured

A simple blood test is all that is needed to find out your A1C. This can be done in a lab or even right in your healthcare provider's office. You don't have to fast the night before to have your A1C checked, either.

How Often It Should Be Checked

Have your A1C checked between two and four times each year. Talk to your healthcare provider about how often you need it checked.

A1C Goals

Joslin Diabetes Center and the American Diabetes Association recommend that most people aim for an A1C below 7%. Ask your doctor or healthcare provider what is best for you.

The results from a large study called the United Kingdom Prospective Diabetes Study (UKPDS) showed that lowering A1C by only 1% lowers the risk of getting complications by 21%!

Taking Action to Lower Your A1C

If your A1C is above your target, talk with your provider and healthcare team about making an action plan to lower it. There are several things you can do to lower your A1C:

- Be more active. Try to do some kind of physical activity most days of the week.

- Follow a healthy eating plan. If you don't have one or aren't sure what to eat, meet with a registered dietitian.

- Check your blood glucose with your meter more often. Your glucose readings will help you and your provider make any needed changes to your treatment plan.

- Change your diabetes medicines. Over time, your diabetes will change, and this means that your medicines will likely have to change, too.

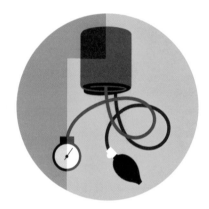

Blood Pressure

People with diabetes are more than twice as likely to have high blood pressure than people without diabetes. High blood pressure is a problem because, if left untreated, it can damage the large vessels leading to your heart and brain and put you at higher risk for heart attack and stroke. For people with diabetes, the goal is a blood pressure lower than 130/80. You will notice that this goal is lower than the target set for most people without diabetes, which is less than 140/90. This is because people with diabetes have a higher risk for heart attack, stroke and heart disease than people without diabetes.

Blood pressure is the force that moves blood through the body. Think of blood pressure as water moving through a hose. When you turn the faucet on low, a gentle force is created, which is what low or normal blood pressure is like. If you turn the faucet on all the way, a strong force is created, similar to what high blood pressure is like. Blood pressure that is high and stays high is called high blood pressure or hypertension.

Why Blood Pressure Is Important

If you have high blood pressure that's not treated, your heart and arteries could be seriously damaged, raising your risk of having a heart attack or stroke or getting kidney disease. By having your blood pressure checked often, you can catch any problems before they can do great harm. Making some lifestyle changes and taking medication can cut the risk of serious heart problems.

How It's Measured

Blood pressure is measured at your healthcare provider's office with a special cuff and a stethoscope. Some people measure their blood pressure at home with a home blood pressure monitor.

How Often It Should Be Checked

Try to have your blood pressure checked every time you see your healthcare team. But make sure your blood pressure is checked at least once a year. You can't feel whether or not your pressure is high, so you may not think it's important to get it checked, but it is! Blood pressure machines in the grocery store or drug store are not very reliable, so these don't count. If you have high blood pressure, talk to your provider about getting a home blood pressure monitor and how often you should check your own blood pressure.

> **Ask what your blood pressure number is at every visit.**

Blood Pressure Goals

For most people with diabetes, the goal for blood pressure is less than 130/80. Your goal depends on certain factors, however, such as whether you also have heart disease or kidney disease. People with kidney disease may have a lower blood pressure goal, such as less than 125/75. Find out your goal from your provider, and remember that both your top and bottom numbers should be at or under your target.

Taking Action to Lower Your Blood Pressure

Once you know what your blood pressure goal is, you can take steps to reach your goal if your blood pressure is too high.

- Have your blood pressure checked at every office visit and keep track of your numbers.
- Be active. Walk for 30 to 60 minutes every day, or find another type of activity that you enjoy and will stay with.
- Eat more fruits, vegetables, whole grains and lowfat dairy foods.
- Cut back on sodium (found in most canned and packaged foods) and limit or avoid adding salt to foods.
- Aim to be at a weight that's healthy for you. Losing even 5 to 10 pounds can help lower your blood pressure as well as your blood glucose.
- If you smoke, talk to your healthcare provider about ways to quit.

- Go easy with alcohol. If you're a man, limit alcohol to no more than two drinks per day; if you're a woman, no more than 1 drink per day.

- Lower stress. Everyone has stress, but there are ways to manage it. Try deep breathing exercises, learn to meditate or take a yoga class. Seek help if stress becomes hard for you to manage.

- If you have high blood pressure, buy a home blood pressure cuff and check it at home regularly.

- You may need to take medicine if lifestyle changes aren't enough to get your blood pressure down to goal. Have a talk with your healthcare provider about taking medication to lower it. (Some people need to take several different types of blood pressure pills to get their blood pressure to target.) The good news is that many blood pressure medicines can also help your heart and kidneys.

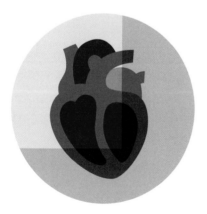

Cholesterol and Triglycerides (Lipids)

Cholesterol and fat that are in your blood are called lipids. Some lipids are good, some are bad. The body needs some lipids to stay healthy, but too much of the wrong type of lipids can damage blood vessels and cause a heart attack or stroke.

> **HDL is good cholesterol.**
> **LDL is bad cholesterol.**

Cholesterol is made by your liver, but it also comes from certain foods. There are two main types of cholesterol: HDL, or "good" cholesterol, which can protect against heart disease, and LDL or "bad" cholesterol, which can raise your risk of heart disease.

Triglycerides, which are fats, come from food, but are also found in the body. Triglycerides are needed for energy; however, if the amount in the blood gets too high, they too can raise your risk of having a heart attack.

Why Lipids Are Important

Knowing what your lipid numbers are can help you to know how well your heart and blood vessels are working. This is important because having diabetes puts you at high risk for heart attack and stroke.

How They're Measured

Lipids are measured by a blood test done at your provider's office or at a lab. If you are having your triglycerides measured, you should fast (not eat anything) for at least 8 hours before the test.

How Often They Should Be Checked

Have your lipids checked at least once a year. If your LDL cholesterol or triglycerides are high, your provider may check them more often.

Lipid Goals

There are three numbers to remember when you have your lipids checked:

- LDL: Less than 100, or less than 70 if you already have heart disease or have had a heart attack
- HDL: Higher than 40 if you're a man, and higher than 50 if you're a woman
- Triglycerides: Less than 150

Taking Action to Reach Lipid Goals

If your LDL is too high:

- Meet with a dietitian for a heart-healthy eating plan.
- Cut back on red meat, and eat more poultry and fish.
- Eat fish and seafood (not fried) at least twice each week.
- Switch to nonfat or lowfat milk and yogurt.
- Use a trans fat-free vegetable oil spread in place of stick margarine or butter.
- Cook with olive, canola or corn oil.
- Bake, broil, grill or poach foods instead of frying.
- Eat more meatless meals made with tofu or legumes (beans, chickpeas, lentils).
- Eat oatmeal, oat bran, fruits and vegetables for soluble fiber, which can help lower LDL cholesterol.
- Limit fatty snack foods such as cookies, potato chips, and some crackers.
- Ask your provider if a cholesterol-lowering medicine, called a statin, can help.

If your HDL is too low:

- Be more active. Aim to do some kind of physical activity, such as walking, most days of the week.
- If you smoke, make a plan to stop.
- Lose weight if you need to. For every 6 pounds you lose, you may be able to increase your HDL by one point.
- Use heart-healthy fats, such as olive and canola oil, on foods and in cooking.

If your triglycerides are too high:

- Cut back on refined carbohydrate foods, such as sugar, sweets, juice, white bread, white pasta and white rice. Choose whole-grain foods, instead.
- Eat less saturated fat, found in red meat, cheese and butter.
- Eat foods that contain omega-3 fatty acids, such as fatty fish (for example, salmon or tuna), walnuts and flaxseed.
- Aim to get your glucose and A1C levels to your target.
- Work on reaching a healthy weight for you.

> **Call your healthcare provider if you have pains in your chest, neck or arms or if you have a hard time breathing. If you can't reach your healthcare provider right away, call 911.**

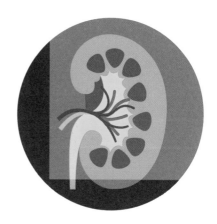

Microalbumin and eGFR (estimated glomerular filtration rate)

Having diabetes means you are at higher risk for serious kidney problems. It is possible for kidney damage to occur after many years of having high A1C levels (above 7%) or high blood glucose levels. (Occasional high blood glucose levels will not cause kidney disease.) Having this simple urine test, called the microalbumin test, done each year can help catch any problems early on. Proper treatment can stop or slow the problems before they become serious.

A microalbumin test looks for very small amounts of a protein called albumin in the urine. Albumin can leak into the urine if the kidneys are damaged. The microalbumin test is the best way to spot signs of early kidney damage and allow treatment to begin that can prevent more serious problems down the road.

The eGFR is another test that tells how well your kidneys are working. Your healthcare provider can calculate this number with a simple blood test that measures creatinine, a substance that comes from muscles. The eGFR measures how well your kidneys are filtering creatinine out of your blood.

Why They're Important

These two tests are important because they provide very early warning signs about changes in your kidney health. When problems are caught in the early stages there are very effective approaches to treating them.

How They're Measured

All that's needed for the microalbumin test is a urine sample. This test can be done right in the lab. Make sure you have a microalbumin test done, and not a routine "dipstick" test that many doctor's offices use.

Your provider will calculate your eGFR based on your age, your sex and your race and by using the results from your creatinine test, a simple blood test.

How Often They Should Be Checked

Make sure you have a microalbumin test done at least once a year.

The eGFR should also be checked at least once a year. You may need to have it checked more often if your kidneys are not working as well as they should.

Microalbumin and eGFR Goals

The goal for the microalbumin test is to have a result of 30 mg or lower. If the result is higher, have it rechecked two or three times within the next 3–6 months. There are other reasons besides diabetes that may cause a high reading, such as pregnancy, a urinary tract infection, menstrual bleeding, or doing a lot of exercise. If the reading is 30–299 mg, it indicates early-stage kidney disease. If the reading is 300 mg or higher, it means the kidney disease is more advanced.

An eGFR result lower than 60 ml/min may indicate early kidney disease.

Taking Action to Reduce the Risk of Kidney Disease

You can do several things to slow or stop kidney problems, especially if you catch the problems early enough:

- Keep your A1C and blood glucose in target range as much as possible.

- Keep your blood pressure at or below your target goal. For most people with diabetes, the goal for blood pressure is less than 130/80.

- Talk to your doctor about taking an ACE inhibitor or an ARB. These are medicines that can keep your microalbumin from rising. They can also help control blood pressure.

- If you smoke or use tobacco products, try to quit.

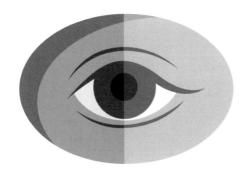

Eye Exam

The best way to avoid eye problems, including loss of vision, is to have regular eye exams.

What It Is

People with diabetes should have a dilated eye exam so the doctor can see the area in the back of the eye where the retina is located.

Why It's Important

Studies show that having regular dilated eye exams by an eye doctor experienced in diabetes can find any eye problems early so they can be successfully treated and sometimes even reversed.

How It's Done

An experienced eye doctor, usually an ophthalmologist, will put special drops in your eyes to open up your pupils. This allows the doctor to see the retina in the back of each of your eyes with a special magnifying lens. Your doctor will also check the pressure in your eyes and will have you read from an eye chart.

How Often It Should Be Done

You should have a dilated eye exam at least once each year. You may need eye exams more often if you have signs of diabetic eye disease, called retinopathy. If your eye doctor finds signs of macular edema, glaucoma or cataracts, you may need other types of tests to determine how to best treat these conditions.

Eye Exam Goals

Unlike A1C, blood pressure or lipids, there is no special number to aim for with an eye exam. The goal is simple: no retinopathy or other eye problems. If you do have retinopathy, your eye doctor will tell you what kind, or stage, you have. Early stages of retinopathy may not need treatment, but if it advances, laser therapy may be needed. Untreated retinopathy and macular edema can lead to vision loss but, luckily, these two conditions can be treated if caught early.

Taking Action to Prevent Eye Disease

As with most complications, you can lessen your chances of developing diabetes eye problems by:

- keeping your A1C and blood glucose within target range

- keeping your blood pressure below 130/80

- having a dilated eye exam at least once every year

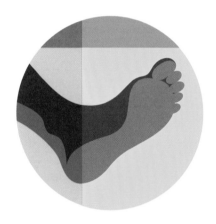

Foot Exam

People with diabetes have a greater chance of developing foot problems than people without diabetes. Left untreated, nerve damage and problems with circulation can result.

While you may be checking your feet at home (hopefully every day!), your provider will also do a more thorough foot exam during one of your regular office visits.

Why It's Important

Nerve damage, called neuropathy, is a common problem for people with diabetes. It can lead to a loss of feeling in the feet, and this can lead to injury or infection. Also, diabetes may cause blood vessels to narrow in the legs and feet, leading to poor circulation. This, in turn, may cause cramps in the legs, slow-healing cuts, lack of normal hair growth and pain in the legs and feet. Poor circulation puts you at risk for infections, as well. Foot infections are very serious if they are not treated in time, and can lead to loss of a toe or even a foot.

How It's Done

During a foot exam, your provider will look at your feet for any skin color changes, cuts, sores or infections. She will check your pulse in certain places on your foot to check your circulation. Finally, she will check the feeling in your feet using a tuning fork or a small plastic wire called a monofilament.

How Often It Should Be Done

Your provider should do a foot exam at least once a year. You may need a foot exam more often if you already have neuropathy, poor circulation, are prone to foot infections, or if you smoke. Help remind your provider to check your feet by removing your shoes and socks or stockings in the exam room.

Foot Exam Goals

Just as with your eye exam, the goal for your foot exam is: no problems! This means that you have no loss of sensation or circulation and no cuts, sores or infections.

Taking Action to Prevent Foot Problems

You can do a lot to avoid foot problems:

- Check your feet every day. Look for areas of redness, dryness, or breaks in the skin, especially around the toenails and between the toes. Call your provider if you notice sores or infections that do not seem to be healing properly. Redness, swelling and increased warmth are usually signs of infection. If you can't bend down to see your feet, use a hand mirror or purchase a special mirror that allows you to see the bottoms of your feet. If your vision is impaired, ask someone to check your feet for you.

- Wash your feet every day in warm soapy water. Don't soak them, and avoid using hot water. Use a mild soap. Dry your feet carefully, especially between your toes.

- After washing and drying your feet, apply a moisturizing lotion that doesn't contain perfumes. Avoid putting lotion between your toes. If your feet perspire, use talcum or baby powder, but not between your toes.

- File your toenails with an emery board. Never use scissors or clippers. Don't file your nails shorter than the ends of your toes. If you have impaired vision, circulation problems, ingrown toenails or fungal nail infections, see a foot doctor called a podiatrist.

- Wear proper-fitting shoes and socks.

- Tell your provider if you have any pain, tingling or loss of feeling in your legs, feet or fingers.

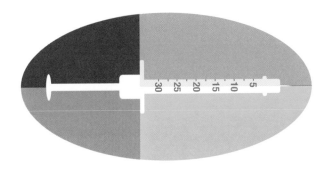

Immunizations

When you have diabetes, it's important to keep up to date with vaccinations, or immunizations. Vaccines can prevent certain illnesses that can be very serious for people with diabetes.

Two of the most important vaccines to get are the influenza, or flu, vaccine and the pneumonia, or pneumococcal, vaccine. Your provider may recommend other vaccinations as well, such as vaccines to prevent herpes zoster, tetanus and hepatitis A and B.

The flu and the pneumonia vaccines are given as injections, usually at your provider's office, a community clinic, or your local pharmacy.

Why They're Important

The flu is a serious illness that can lead to pneumonia and even death. People with diabetes can become very ill when they get the flu and may need to be hospitalized. Getting a flu shot doesn't guarantee that you won't get the flu, but you're less likely to get it for about six months after getting the vaccine. Pneumonia is also a serious illness that affects the lungs and may also lead to infections of the blood and the covering of the brain (meningitis).

How Often

It's recommended that people with diabetes get the flu vaccine every year. The best time to get the flu shot is during September, October or November, before the flu season begins. You can get a pneumonia shot at any time of the year, including when you get your flu shot. For most people, one pneumonia shot is enough for life. But if you're under age 65, ask your provider if you should get another pneumonia shot 5–10 years after getting the first one.

Taking Action

- Make a note on your calendar to get your flu shot every year.
- Get a pneumonia vaccine if you haven't already had one.
- Talk to your provider about other immunizations that you may need, especially if you will be traveling.

> **If you smoke, make a plan to quit—TODAY.**

Stop Smoking

People with diabetes should not smoke. Smoking damages the blood vessels and raises the risk of heart disease, not to mention other diseases.

Why It's Important

Smoking, which refers to the use of any type of tobacco product, including pipes, cigars, chewing tobacco and snuff, increases your risk of heart disease, along with lung cancer, stroke, emphysema and foot and leg problems.

It's not always easy to stop smoking, but it can be done! Talk to your provider about ways to stop smoking. Smoking cessation programs are available, along with medication, patches and nicotine gum to help you quit.

Taking Action

- Make a plan to quit smoking. Set a "quit date" and let your family and friends know so that they can help you.
- Make a list of reasons to stop smoking and refer to it often.
- Throw away cigarettes, tobacco, matches and ashtrays.
- Find out about local classes and support groups in your area.
- Talk with your provider about whether medications, hypnosis or even acupuncture might be helpful for you.
- Set goals for yourself and reward yourself when you achieve them.

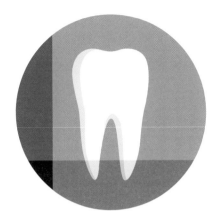

Dental Exam

Oral health refers to the health of your mouth, teeth and gums. Because diabetes can affect your oral health, taking care of both your oral health and your diabetes can help prevent problems with your gums and teeth.

Why It's Important

Diabetes can make it harder for your body, including your gums, to fight off infections. Poorly controlled blood glucose levels can cause the following oral problems:

- gingivitis or periodontitis
- tooth loss
- thrush, a fungal infection in the mouth
- dry mouth

Periodontal disease (PD) can increase blood glucose levels and increase the amount of insulin that you need. It can also be more difficult to treat PD when you have diabetes, especially if your glucose levels are high.

See your dentist at least twice a year and make sure that he or she knows that you have diabetes.

Taking Action

- Aim to keep your A1C and blood glucose levels within your target range.
- See your dentist at least a twice a year.
- Brush your teeth twice a day and floss once a day.
- Call your dentist if you have any signs of PD, including bleeding or swollen gums, separating or loosening teeth, or gums that have pulled away from the teeth.
- Be physically active and eat healthfully.
- If you smoke, stop.

The Best Care

In order to get the best diabetes care, you need to know what that "best care" looks like. That is, you should know which lab tests and exams you should have each year in order to be sure that everything that can be done to manage your diabetes is being done. Just in case your provider forgets, you should give a friendly reminder. Don't forget to ask about the results of the tests, and what the results mean for you.

If you take insulin, the usual recommendation is to see your doctor about your diabetes four times a year. If you take pills, or if your diabetes is controlled by a meal plan and physical activity, your doctor may recommend that you only need to be seen every six months. It is a good idea to talk to a diabetes educator about once a year to determine if there is any new information you need to know to help you manage your diabetes.

Tests, Goals and Results

Below is a helpful chart which you should use to record information about your goals and your results.

Tests	Usual Goal	Your Target	Results			
			Date	Date	Date	Date
Blood pressure at every visit or 2–4 times a year	Less than 130/80					
Total cholesterol once a year	Less than 200					
LDL cholesterol once a year	Less than 100					
HDL cholesterol once a year	Greater than 40 (men) Greater than 50 (women)					
Triglycerides once a year	Less than 150					
Micro-albuminuria once a year	Less than 30					
Eye exam	Once a year					
A1C two – four times a year	Less than 7					
Dental exam twice a year	Early detection					
Foot exam at every visit	Early detection					

Chapter 11
Living with Diabetes

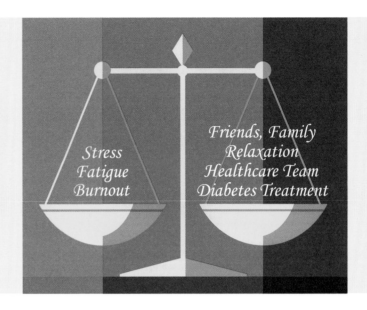

Stress
Fatigue
Burnout

Friends, Family
Relaxation
Healthcare Team
Diabetes Treatment

Riding the Emotional Roller Coaster

If you have diabetes, you have a wide range of special challenges. The first of these challenges concerns your physical well-being. You have to learn how your body works, how it uses the food you eat for energy, and how your diabetes affects it. Other challenges you face are emotional. You need to cope with how diabetes makes you feel–and how you feel about having diabetes. Emotional reactions, stress and depression can all have an effect on blood glucose control. Living with diabetes involves thinking about how to involve family members, loved ones, friends and coworkers. It involves anticipating, problem-solving and planning ahead. This chapter addresses the emotional ups and downs of having diabetes and offers tips for steps to take to live well with diabetes.

To succeed with diabetes, it is important that you understand the difficult thoughts and feelings that may arise. First, recognize that feeling upset about diabetes is quite normal. Most people go through times when they feel distressed about living with diabetes. On occasion, this has to do with the day-to-day frustrations of the illness itself, which can be

annoying, burdensome and confusing. At other times, your feelings about having diabetes can become overwhelming. These can include:

- anger ("Why me? This isn't fair!")
- fear ("What is going to happen to me? Am I doomed?")
- guilt ("I must have done something to deserve this! If only I hadn't been eating all those sweet things!")
- depression ("I feel so alone and defeated by all this!")
- denial ("I can just ignore diabetes; this is no big deal.").

It's completely normal to have some or all of these feelings. These feelings tend to lessen as you learn to live and cope with having diabetes.

The good news is that there is a lot you can do to deal with the feelings that you have. Here are some ideas:

- Talk to family or friends about what is bothering you.
- Join a diabetes support group.
- Find a time each day for a bit of quiet relaxation.

- To avoid feeling overwhelmed by diabetes, make sure that you have a plan for self-management that is clear and reasonable for you. If you are confused, don't be shy—ask questions!

By becoming more actively involved in your diabetes management, you will feel more confident about your own abilities, less angry and fearful about diabetes, and more motivated to keep up your efforts.

Stress, Depression and Diabetes Control

The stresses and emotions of everyday life can negatively affect your diabetes. For some, stress may directly influence blood glucose levels. For others, the influence may be more indirect. For example, it may make it difficult to give your diabetes treatment routine the necessary time and attention.

You may find that stress can either raise or lower blood glucose levels. When stress hormones (such as the fight-or-flight hormone, adrenaline) are released in your body blood glucose levels go up. On the other hand, when you face stressful or emotional situations, you may change certain routine behaviors, which can make your glucose levels fluctuate. For example, you may skip meals, causing glucose levels to drop, or you may overeat, causing them to rise.

There are a lot of ways to manage stress. Remember that everyone has stress in their lives and it probably won't go away. It's how you deal with stress that's important. Things that can help include:

- eating healthfully and getting regular physical activity
- making time to do activities that you enjoy
- learning how to relax through deep breathing, visualization, meditation or yoga
- talking to family, friends or a counselor

People with diabetes are more likely to be depressed than people without diabetes. This is because taking care of diabetes is often complex, demanding, and frustrating. Depression is common among people with type 1 and type 2 diabetes, people with poor blood glucose control, and those suffering from complications due to diabetes. Why? If you consider that a feeling of helplessness is one of the most common causes of depression, it is easy to understand how the frustration and unpredictability of blood glucose control could lead to feeling helpless despite one's best efforts.

How do you know if you might be depressed? The main difference between serious or "clinical" depression and common sadness or grief is in its time and intensity. Clinical depression is more than the normal response of feeling down for a couple of hours or days. It

Depression is not recognized often enough, which is unfortunate, because when it is diagnosed, good treatments are available.

is more dramatic and it takes you down farther and longer. Ask yourself how often over the last 2 weeks have you felt:

- depressed when you think about living with diabetes?
- little interest or joy in the activities of your life?
- helpless about the ability to make any positive changes with your diabetes treatment plan?

If you have felt any of these symptoms most of the day, nearly every day, during the last 2 weeks, then consider depression as a possible explanation. Talk with your healthcare provider if you think you may be depressed. Your provider may refer you to counseling with a mental health specialist, and/or prescribe medication.

You can do other things to improve your mood such as:

- Push yourself to be with other people rather than alone.
- Seek support from family and friends.
- Join a diabetes support group (online or in person).
- Prioritize self-care changes that you need to make.
- Limit making changes to one change at a time.
- Remember what helped before with similar problems.
- Find spiritual support, if appropriate.

Involving Others: How Family and Friends Can Help

As much as possible, talk to your family and friends about your diabetes. Share this book. Bring them with you to a diabetes education class. The more they know and understand about your daily routine for caring for your diabetes, the more they can be helpful. In some cases, you'll need to tell them what to do if your blood glucose goes too low or if other kinds of emergency action may be needed. You may want to teach certain people in your life how to give an injection or take a blood glucose reading. Certainly, you don't need to let everyone know you have diabetes if you don't want to. But the more you talk about it, the more you may find support from others who have it too.

At the same time, sometimes family and friends try to be too helpful. They may end up being "misguided helpers." A misguided helper is the person whom you feel is overly monitoring your every move with statements like "should you be eating THAT?" or "don't you think you should check your blood glucose?" Let your loved ones know what kinds of statements you find helpful and encouraging, when you want them to stand back and when you don't mind them stepping in with helpful statements of support (such as, "would you like to join me for a walk later today?)

Ten Tips: Keys to Success for Managing Diabetes

The following list highlights tips that can help you deal with your diabetes. Review this list on a regular basis, refocusing your feelings and thoughts as other circumstances in your life change.

1. Set realistic, achievable goals and expectations for yourself and for your diabetes

- Make a list of some "quick to fix" goals. For example, check blood glucose 2 hours after supper, or change all sodas to diet soda.
- Set a date and time to check progress and add new goals.

2. Monitor your progress

- Keep a diary of your progress and slips on a daily basis. Slips are normal and to be expected. Research shows that people who routinely monitor their progress are more likely to maintain weight loss and fitness goals.
- Don't try to do everything at once. Make changes gradually.
- Learn from what has worked for you in the past and do it again!

3. Plan ahead: What will make it easier for you to stick to your diabetes plan?

- Plan for high-risk situations (such as parties) where you are likely to slip.
- Give yourself a variety of choices and alternatives that might work.
- Contact support people you can trust—family, friends, spouses, coworkers.
- Join clubs or support groups and tell them what you need.
- List ways to reward yourself and praise yourself for positive changes, rather than berate yourself for slips.

4. Be aware of the stumbling blocks

- Identify barriers that can make it hard to take care of your diabetes. Are you tempted to eat second portions of food? Is it hard to check your blood glucose at work or school?
- By focusing on major stumbling blocks to your diabetes care, you can find ways around them.

5. Learning about diabetes is lifelong

- Treatments for diabetes are constantly improving based on new research. Stay informed.
- Learn as much as you can about meal planning, physical activity, medications and reducing risks for complications. Bring questions to your healthcare provider to discuss.

6. Manage stress and your emotional health

- Pay attention to factors in your life that cause tension, wear you down or make you anxious. Work with your healthcare team to reduce these stresses.

- Recognize early signs of depression and talk with your healthcare provider.

7. Be prepared

- Unlike people who don't have diabetes, you may have to plan aspects of your day. Also, you need to be ready to handle high and low blood glucose levels. Being prepared can help you feel more at ease and in control.

- Practice problem-solving. Ask yourself what if.... (I forget my medicine; I eat too much; I get sick; my blood glucose goes too high/low) and know how to respond ahead of an emergency.

- Remember that you can continue to do the things that you liked to do before you got diabetes.

8. Be realistic

- You're not always going to be in perfect control of your diabetes. You will have good days and bad days. That's okay.

- When you occasionally have a bad day, don't dwell on it. Simply try to continue without guilt or blame. The goal is to do the best that you can, and accept that no one is perfect.

9. Ask for support

- Tell your family and friends that you appreciate their support. Let them know what is and isn't helpful to you (something that is supportive to one person may not be supportive to another).

- Tell family and friends specific ways they can help you follow your treatment program.

10. Build a healthcare team

- You don't have to do it alone. Doctors, nurses and nurse practitioners, diabetes educators and behavioral specialists can help you solve the tough problems and feel more confident about caring for your diabetes.

Notes and Reminders

_____

_____

_____

_____

_____

_____

_____

_____

_____

_____

_____

_____

_____

Chapter 12
Pregnancy

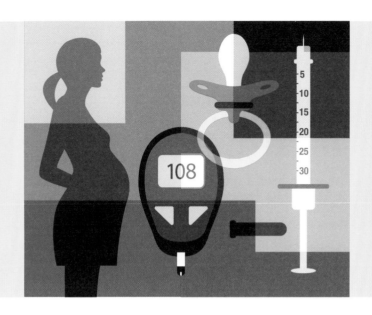

Planning and Managing for a Successful Pregnancy

Imagine wanting to get pregnant and being discouraged from doing so. About 25 years ago this was the case for many women with diabetes. But fortunately, with recent advances in diabetes management, and with careful planning, the chances of having a successful pregnancy are excellent!

Preconception Planning

If you have diabetes and are thinking about becoming pregnant, it is recommended that you start preparing about 6 months prior to conception. The most important thing to do before conception is to have your diabetes in good control and to learn how to continue managing your diabetes during pregnancy. Schedule a talk early with your healthcare provider. He or she will help you get ready for pregnancy.

Once you've decided you want to become pregnant, you should make an appointment with your endocrinologist (a diabetes physician specialist) to review your health status and pregnancy plans. If you don't have an endocrinologist, your primary care provider can refer you to one. In addition to the endocrinologist, there are others who can help you during your pregnancy: an obstetrician, of course; but other members of your healthcare team may include a nurse who focuses on the management of diabetes, a registered dietitian, and an ophthalmologist who will be sure your eyes stay healthy. While you will be the one in charge of your pregnancy, it is still necessary to have a medical team as well as loved ones to support you during this time.

You will need to meet with your obstetrician more frequently than a woman without diabetes. These visits may include ultrasounds to determine fetal growth and development) and other laboratory tests. It is important to know that you will be scheduling a number of visits with your team during pregnancy.

Prepregnancy Checklist

Before you decide to become pregnant, make sure you can answer "yes" to the following:

- your blood glucose is in good control (A1C less than 7% or as near normal as possible)

- your blood pressure is under control (below 130/80 mm Hg, and if you are taking medication for your blood pressure, the medicine is safe for use when pregnant)

- you are familiar with and comfortable with the skills needed for diabetes self-management (blood glucose monitoring, meal planning, taking medication, target blood glucose levels, etc.)

- you have identified a pregnancy healthcare team

- you have completed a prepregnancy health check-up, including a dilated eye exam

Blood Glucose Control

The critical stages of development for a baby begin within the first 8 weeks, which is often when a woman can't even tell she is pregnant. Even so, during this time the baby's spine and organs are formed. This is why it is extremely important to have your blood glucose under control prior to conception in order to help reduce the risk of harm to the baby. Checking your blood glucose daily and having an A1C test will help tell you if you're staying on track. During your pregnancy your A1C is typically checked every month.

Prepregnancy Blood Glucose Goals

Measurement	Goal
Fasting and before meals	80–110 mg/dl
1 hour after meals	100–155 mg/dl
2 hours after meals	100–145 mg/dl
A1C	Less than 7% and as close to 6% as possible without resulting in hypoglycemia

If You Are Already Pregnant

More than half of all pregnancies are unplanned. If you into fall into this category, once you discover that you are pregnant, it's important that you schedule an appointment with your diabetes healthcare team and your obstetrician right away.

Glucose Control

For the health of you and your baby, it's important to achieve the best possible blood glucose control, while avoiding hypoglycemia. Refer to the table below to determine what the recommended glucose goals are when you are pregnant.

> **Keeping your blood glucose and A1C at your targets can help you have a healthy baby.**

Recommended Blood Glucose and Ketone Goals during Pregnancy

Measurement	Goal
Fasting and before meals	60–99 mg/dl
1 hour after meals	100–129 mg/dl
Overnight (2-4 a.m.)	60–99 mg/dl
A1C – 1st trimester	Below 7% and as close to 6% as possible without causing significant hypoglycemia
A1C – 2nd and 3rd trimesters	Below 6%
Urine ketones	Negative

Taking Insulin

Women with type 1 diabetes must take insulin to manage their diabetes, and during pregnancy will find that the dose of insulin will be increased. Because diabetes pills have not been approved by the Food and Drug Administration (FDA) for use during pregnancy, women with type 2 diabetes may also need to take insulin during their pregnancy. As pregnancy progresses, more insulin may be needed to compensate for placental hormones that raise blood glucose; and towards the end, you may need 2–3 times more insulin than you needed before pregnancy. Your healthcare team will work with you to find the insulin combination and dosing that best meets your needs.

Nutrition

You've probably heard the saying that pregnant women are eating for two! The food you eat during pregnancy not only helps the baby grow, but it also has an effect on your blood glucose levels. As mentioned above, a dietitian is an important member of your healthcare team, and part of the dietitian's job will be to provide you with a meal plan that takes into account your and your baby's nutrition needs, your lifestyle, and the foods you like and dislike. A dietitian will be able to tell you which foods are important to eat and which ones you should stay away from, as well as how much weight gain is appropriate for each trimester (3-month period) of your pregnancy.

Activity

It's okay to continue most activities during your pregnancy; however, it is best to check with your healthcare team, especially if the activity is strenuous (like skiing, or long-distance hiking).

Gestational Diabetes

Gestational diabetes is the term used when diabetes is diagnosed during pregnancy. The treatment, blood glucose monitoring, scheduled office visits, meal planning, activity and medication are similar to the guidelines described above. Your healthcare team will help develop a specific care plan for you. It is very important that, once you deliver your baby, you schedule a follow-up appointment for laboratory testing and healthcare review with your healthcare team, because women who have gestational diabetes are at risk for developing type 2 diabetes later on.

Postpartum (After Pregnancy)

After your baby is born and you have seen your obstetrician for a follow-up visit, plan a healthcare check-up visit with your endocrinologist to review your blood glucose control, possible medication changes and weight management.

Chapter 13
Managing Diabetes When You're Older (Over 70)

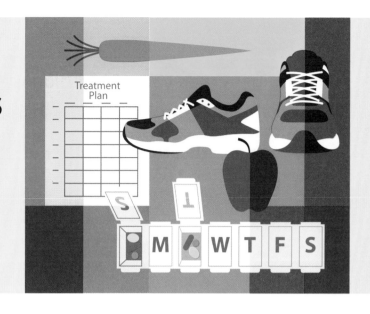

How Managing Your Diabetes Is Different When You're Older

If you are an older adult with diabetes, the treatment is not much different than that for a younger person with diabetes. The goal is to improve the quality and length of your life by preventing or slowing the onset or progression of diabetes complications. Diabetes that is not well-controlled can speed up the progression of complications and interact with other issues related to aging. So, a key goal is to maintain your glucose and A1C levels as close to target as possible, while making sure that you stay safe. Diabetes can be challenging to manage no matter how old you are. Even if you're fairly new to diabetes and don't have any complications, you may have other health conditions that can make it more difficult to manage your diabetes.

Other factors such as your living situation, eating problems and difficulty staying active can make it harder to manage diabetes. The good news is that there are a lot of ways to make living with diabetes easier: specially trained people, medicines and medical devices and resources that you can call on for special help.

You can live a long, healthy life with diabetes, but you may need to make some changes in your diabetes treatment plan so that you stay healthy.

A1C and Blood Glucose Goals

- The usual goal for A1C is less than 7%
- The usual goal for blood glucose is:
    - 70–130 before meals
    - less than 180 two hours after meals
    - 90–150 before bedtime

The best way to know how your diabetes treatment plan is working is to have your A1C checked every 3 to 6 months and to check your blood glucose at home with your meter. Your blood glucose and A1C targets may stay the same as you get older or they may be higher depending on the other health problems you have. It is important not to let blood glucose levels go too high (which can put you at risk for increased infections, worsen any diabetes complications you may have or make you feel unwell), or too low (putting you at risk for confusion, possible falls and injury). Talk to your healthcare provider about what the A1C and blood glucose targets are for you.

> As you get older, your blood glucose and A1C goals may be set higher if you have other serious health problems.
>
> Ask your healthcare provider what your A1C and blood glucose should be.

Remember:

- As you get older, your blood glucose and A1C goals may be set higher if you have other serious health problems.
- Ask your healthcare provider what your A1C and blood glucose should be.

Checking Your Blood Glucose

- Talk to your healthcare provider about how often to check your blood glucose. This can vary depending on what diabetes medicines you take.
- Let your provider know if you are having problems using your meter, reading the numbers or getting a drop of blood. Some meters are easier to use than others, and there are meters with large numbers and even ones that can talk! Your pharmacist or healthcare provider should be able to help you find the meter that's right for you.
- Take your blood glucose numbers with you to your provider's office and ask him or her to review them.

- If you are "feeling funny" or not feeling well, check your blood glucose. Sometimes when your blood glucose is high or low it can make you feel different.

Medications

As you get older, you may find that you have to take several kinds of pills and maybe even insulin for your diabetes, and you may need to take medication for other conditions as well. It can be confusing and stressful trying to keep all of your medications straight and to remember when to take them. Some pills may be hard to swallow, and injecting insulin with a syringe may be difficult if you have arthritis, for example. Here are some tips for making it easier to take your medications:

- Talk with your healthcare provider. Let her know all of the medicines that you're taking. She may be able to adjust or change your medications so that you can control your diabetes in the easiest way possible. Be sure to ask.

> Checking your blood glucose is an important way for you to know how you are doing with your diabetes from day to day. You can't rely on how you are feeling to know what your blood glucose levels are.

- Take all of your medications with you when you see your provider–even those for conditions other than diabetes.

- If you take or need to start taking insulin, premixed insulins are available, as well as insulin pens to make it easier to inject.

- Let your provider know if money is a problem. She may be able to prescribe generic medications. Other resources are also available that can help.

> **Medication reminders and writing down what you have taken is especially important when you take several medicines or are on insulin.**

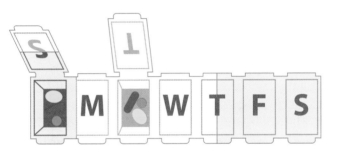

Keeping Track of Medicines

Keeping track by memory of the medicines you have taken can be difficult. Developing a system to help you remember to take your medicines is important.

Here are some useful ways people have found to help them remember their medicines:

- Use a 7-day pill case. Ask someone to fill it for you if you need help.

- As you take each medicine, write it down on a calendar.

- Set alarms as reminders that it's time to take your medicine.

- Keep your pills on your kitchen table or in another place to help you remember to take them.

- Have a family member remind you.

Low Blood Glucose (Hypoglycemia)

Treating low blood glucose, or hypoglycemia, is the same for the older adult as it is for someone who is younger (see Chapter 7). The difference is that as you get older you may not feel your lows as quickly as someone who is younger or you may not feel the symptoms as strongly. This is especially true if you are on a medicine called a beta blocker.

Tips to help keep you safe:

- Check your blood glucose even if you just feel a little funny or dizzy; you could have low blood glucose.

- Always carry a treatment for low blood glucose, such as glucose tablets, with you.

- Let your provider know if you are afraid of having low blood glucose.

- Always check your blood glucose before you drive; if your glucose is less than 100 before driving, have a snack, such as a piece of fruit, some crackers or some yogurt.

- Always check your blood glucose before and after doing physical activity.

- Call your healthcare provider if your blood glucose goes below 70 more than once a week.

Physical Activity

- Staying active is important, not only because it makes you feel good, but also because it can help control your blood glucose, cholesterol, blood pressure and weight. Physical activity can get harder as you get older due to joint problems, back pain and other health issues. You may be afraid of falling or think you can't exercise because you have heart problems. But remember there are many ways that you can stay physically fit at any age.

- Talk to your healthcare provider about the types of activities that you can do safely. Ask for a referral to an exercise physiologist or a physical therapist. They can help you find activities that are safe and enjoyable for you.

- Try to do something active every day, such as walking, gardening, climbing stairs in your home or biking. You might try walking in a shopping mall or joining a community center that offers group classes.

- If you are having trouble with balance or are worried about falling, talk to your provider about seeing a physical therapist.

- If you need a cane or walker to be physically active, use one. It is more important to keep moving safely than it is to avoid using these assistive devices and avoid being active.

- If you are on diabetes medicines that cause low blood glucose, check your blood glucose before and after any activity. If it is an activity that lasts several hours (such as yard work), check your blood glucose every hour during the activity. Always keep a treatment for low blood glucose with you during your activity.

> **Staying active is important at any age and any activity that you do will be helpful.**

Nutrition

When you have diabetes, it's important to eat the foods you like, but also to control the amount of carbohydrates you are eating. This can be challenging at any age, but can grow even more challenging as you get older. Some of the more common problems that older adults have are a lack of appetite, stomach or swallowing problems, problems with chewing due to tooth loss, social isolation and financial issues. Here are some steps you can take to make sure you are the eating as healthfully as you can:

- Ask your healthcare provider to refer you to a dietitian who will help you select foods that you like to eat. A dietitian will also take into account any eating problems that you may have as well as the amount of physical activity that you do.

- Eat a variety of foods and keep an eye on portion sizes. Use the plate method (see Chapter 2) to help you.

- Aim to be at a weight that's healthy for you.

- Eat three meals every day and make sure not to skip meals. Skipping meals can put you at higher risk for low blood glucose levels. If you don't feel like eating, consider using a meal replacement drink made for people who have diabetes. Ask your dietitian or pharmacist about these.

- If you are having problems with your teeth, let your provider or dentist know.

- Make plans to eat with a friend or relative a few times a week or check to see if your local senior center provides meals.

- In many cities and states programs are available, such as Meals on Wheels, that will deliver meals right to your home. If you are on a fixed income, these programs are often offered at a very low cost or may even be free.

You don't have to buy special foods when you have diabetes. Eating a balanced, nutritious meal plan is the most important step you can take.

> **If you are having problems eating enough or are unsure what to do about your meal plan, talk to your provider about meeting with a dietitian.**

Don't Lose Sight of Anything

Poor or failing eyesight, whether caused by a complication of diabetes or some other reason, can make dealing with diabetes more difficult. There are treatments available that may help you improve your vision.

- Make sure to get a dilated eye exam every year.

- Use a magnifier if you are having difficulty seeing your pills or insulin syringe. A diabetes educator or pharmacist can help you with this.

- Talk to your provider about switching to an insulin pen if you cannot see the lines on your insulin syringe

Take Good Care of Your Feet

You may have problems with your feet, such as decreased circulation, lack of feeling or pain.

- Check your feet daily (including the tops and bottoms of your feet and between the toes) for redness, open areas or cracks in the skin.

- Take care of cuts or sores right away and seek help if they are not healing.

- Use lotion for dry skin, but not between the toes.

- If you can't reach your feet, place a mirror against the wall or buy a special mirror with a long handle that will allow you to see the bottoms of your feet. Or ask a family member to help you.

- Don't go barefoot. Wear well-fitting shoes.

- Have a podiatrist clip your nails (Medicare will pay for this).

- If you have problems, such as bunions or hammer toes, Medicare will pay for special diabetic shoes.

- Have your healthcare provider check your feet at every visit. Remove your shoes and socks when you're in the exam room to remind her!

Coping with Diabetes

It can be stressful to live with diabetes, and even more so if you have other health concerns or are the caregiver for someone else in your family. If you are feeling anxious or depressed or just having difficulty doing your daily activities, here are a few things you can do:

- Let your provider know that you are having trouble. He can recommend that you see a diabetes educator or social worker who will have suggestions for making things easier for you.

- If you are feeling depressed, down or sad, tell your provider. Treatment is available to help you.

- Ask your family members or friends for help. This may seem hard to do, but chances are, they'll be happy to help. Let them know what they can do, such as helping you with your medicines, driving you to medical appointments, grocery shopping or even just talking.

- Find out about the services available for older adults in your community, such as rides and homecare services.

- Get plenty of rest and try to keep your blood glucose levels controlled. This will give you the energy you need to cope with life's troubles.

- Break big tasks into little steps, so that you don't get too overwhelmed.

- Talk to others who have diabetes so that you don't feel alone.

- Know that there is a whole team available to help you, including your provider, nurses, dietitians and diabetes educators.

> **Remember you can live a long and happy life with diabetes. Your healthcare team is there to help you.**

Chapter 14
Be Prepared!

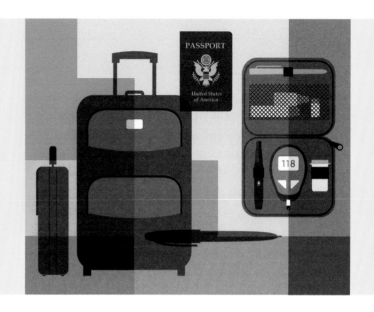

Getting Ready for Your Medical Appointments

Most of the visits with your healthcare provider are probably short. To get the most from your appointments, it's important to have your questions ready and your diabetes information well organized. That way, both you and your provider will learn more that will help you keep track of and manage your diabetes.

Before the Visit: Make Your List and Check It Twice!

Doing a little "homework" before your appointment will help you get the most from your visit.

- Make a list of all of your medications (not just your diabetes medications) as well as any vitamin, mineral or dietary supplements that you take. Note those that need a refill prescription.

- Record blood glucose readings in your log book or download and print out your most recent meter results. Keep in mind that your provider will likely not have time to review a month's worth of results.

- Consider keeping a 3-day food and activity record, and reviewing it with your healthcare team.

- Write down any specific symptoms that you've been having, such as numbness or tingling in your feet.

- Write down any questions that you want answered.

- Be prepared with one or two main issues that you want to focus on and discuss during your visit.

Day of the Visit: Arrive Prepared!

- Take your list of medications and questions, along with your log book, food records and glucose meter.

- Consider inviting a family member or friend along to take notes, listen and be supportive.

During the Visit

- Ask your questions. Make sure you get answers that you understand, and write them down.

- Use the time wisely. Have your list of medications and questions ready, know which prescriptions need refills, ask about your lab and exam results and take your shoes and socks off so that your provider can easily check your feet.

- Ask about other treatment options; things you can do to get your blood glucose, blood pressure and lipids in target; reasons for new medications and their side effects.

After the Visit

- Follow up with your provider to find out results of any lab tests or exams that were done.

- Write down your results to help you keep track.

- Call your provider or diabetes educator if you have questions.

Your Diabetes Healthcare Team

You'll have an easier time taking care of your diabetes if you have a healthcare team to support you. Here's a list of those you might enlist to be on your team:

- your primary care provider; he or she can refer you to specialists, as needed

- an endocrinologist, a doctor who specializes in diabetes

- a diabetes nurse educator, a nurse who can teach you skills needed to manage your diabetes

- a registered dietitian, an expert in food and nutrition who can help you with meal planning and teach you how your food choices affect blood glucose

- an exercise physiologist, a person trained in the science of exercise who can help you develop a safe and effective physical activity program

- a pharmacist, an expert who can help you keep track of all of your medications and explain how they work

- a mental health provider, a social worker, psychologist or psychiatrist who can teach you coping skills, help with behavior change and provide emotional support

Planning for Travel

Whether you're driving across the country or flying off to an exotic locale, traveling, for many people, is one of the highlights of their lives. Luckily, having diabetes doesn't need to stop you from going camping, visiting friends and relatives or taking a cruise. With careful planning, you can take care of your diabetes while traveling just as well as you manage it at home.

If you're thinking about taking a trip, plan as far ahead as possible. Once you know where you're going, how you're getting there, and how long you'll be staying, you can make the following preparations.

1. See your healthcare provider at least four weeks ahead of time to be sure that your general health is okay and that your diabetes is in good control.

> Check your blood glucose more often than usual when you're traveling.

> **Always carry extra diabetes supplies and prescriptions when you travel.**

2. Get a letter from your doctor that says you have diabetes. You may need it if you are ever asked about the supplies, such as syringes, and any medicines you have with you. It's also helpful to have your doctor describe any other conditions or complications that you have in case another doctor needs to take care of you while you're away.

3. Get prescriptions for syringes or pens and pen needles and any medicines you use. You will need them if you lose yours. Carry them with you at all times. Ask your doctor to use the generic names of medications because brand names can vary from country to country.

4. Also ask your doctor for medications to prevent motion sickness and diarrhea.

5. If you are traveling to certain parts of the world, you may need particular immunizations before you go. Find out what you'll need and allow plenty of time to get them. You may need several shots over a period of several months, so plan ahead. It's also a good idea to find out which immunizations you've already had. Keep a record of your immunizations, too.

6. Your doctor may be able to give you the name of a doctor who practices in the area that you plan to visit. If not, contact your local or national office of the American Diabetes Association, which can provide you with names of physicians in those areas. If you're traveling to another country, the International Diabetes Federation can give you the names of diabetes associations in the countries you're visiting. You can also contact the U.S. Embassy in the country you're visiting for names of doctors. Remember, though, that in an emergency, you should go to the nearest hospital.

7. If you'll be traveling across time zones, check with your provider or diabetes educator before leaving. They can help you with when to take your diabetes medicines.

8. If you use an insulin pump, remember that pumps can break and pump supplies may not be readily available away from home. Talk with your provider or diabetes educator about "off-pump" doses of injected insulin to use as a back-up in case your pump breaks while you're traveling. Make sure you carry extra pump supplies with you, too.

9. Plan to take extra supplies of diabetes pills, insulin, syringes or pens and pen needles, meter test strips and any other medications you may need. Take twice as much as you think you'll use in case the place you're visiting doesn't have the supplies you'll need.

10. Make sure you have some type of medical identification to wear or carry with you that states that you have diabetes. This can be a tag that you wear as a bracelet or necklace, or a card that you carry in your wallet that includes an emergency phone number.

11. Make an appointment with your dietitian to discuss when and what to eat if you'll be traveling across time zones. A dietitian can also help you make healthy food choices if you'll be visiting another country.

12. Many airlines no longer serve meals. Call the airline ahead of time to find out if a meal will be served on your flight, what time the meal will be served and what meal options you have. It's a good idea to carry a supply of snacks, such as peanut butter crackers, granola bars, single-serving fruit cups and single-serving boxes of cereal. Also, carry treatment for low blood glucose. Glucose tablets and glucose gel are good choices.

What to Put in Your Travel Bag

When the day comes for you to leave for your trip, include the items listed below in a small travel bag. Keep this bag with you at all times. Don't check the bag on planes, trains or buses; it might get lost. Check with your airline or the Transportation Security Administration (866-289-9673) or www.tsa.gov before you fly to check current regulations about carry-ons.

- Diabetes medicine, including pills, insulin and/or other injectable medicines. If you take insulin, take all the syringes or insulin pens and pen needles that you will need for your trip. Take alcohol to wipe off the tops of the insulin bottles. Do not keep your insulin where it is too cold (below 40

> When you travel make sure you have some type of medical identification to wear or carry with you that states that you have diabetes.

degrees) or too hot (above 86 degrees). If you're traveling to a warm climate, buy a special insulated travel pack that will keep your insulin or other injectable medicines from getting too warm. Remember to bring your travel letter from your doctor that authorizes you to carry these supplies. You may need this letter to get through airport security.

- Glucagon kit if you are at risk for low blood glucose.

- Meter, extra test strips and extra lancets. You may want to take an extra meter or batteries.

- Ketone strips if you take insulin.

- Pump supplies if you use an insulin pump.

- Snacks that contain carbohydrate, such as granola bars or dried fruit, in case of meal delays or low blood glucose.

On the Way

- Carry a card that says you have diabetes. Put your name, address, phone number and your doctor's name and phone number on the card. Put the kind and amount of diabetes medicine you take, and the names of other medicines you use on the card, also. Wear a bracelet or necklace with the same facts on it so that someone can help you if you have a problem.

- Do not skip meals or snacks. Keep snacks with you in case a meal is delayed or you have to miss a meal, or if you have a low blood glucose. Pull off the road if you have a reaction while driving. See chapter 7 for how to prevent and treat low blood glucose.

- While traveling, check your blood glucose more often (at least 3–4 times a day or every 4–6 hours).

- Protect medicine and glucose strips from extreme temperatures by using an insulated case.

- Store medicine and diabetes supplies away from heat and humidity.

- Wear comfortable shoes and socks, and check your feet frequently for blisters; get treatment if even minor foot problems develop.

- Tell people you travel with that you have diabetes and explain how to recognize low blood glucose and how to treat it.

- Do your best to follow your meal plan and physical activity plan as closely as possible.

Diabetes Education

Whether you're newly diagnosed with diabetes or have had diabetes for many years, realize that diabetes education doesn't end. There are always new things to learn about diabetes. Here's how to stay up to date:

- Meet with a certified diabetes educator (CDE). CDEs are usually nurses, dietitians, exercise physiologists and pharmacists who specialize in diabetes education. You can find CDE's working in hospital outpatient departments, medical centers, clinics and physician offices. To find a diabetes educator in your area, visit the American Association of Diabetes Educators (AADE) Web site at www.diabeteseducator.org.

- Meet with a registered dietitian to learn more about diabetes nutrition and meal planning. Many dietitians are also CDEs. Your physician can likely refer you to a dietitian, or you can visit the American Dietetic Association's Web site at www.eatright.org to find a dietitian in your area.

- Attend a diabetes self-management education class. Diabetes classes are usually taught by a CDE and you'll benefit from learning from others in the class, too. To find a diabetes class in your area, contact your local hospital or medical center, or visit the American Diabetes Association's Web site at www.diabetes.org.

- Subscribe to a diabetes magazine, such as *Diabetes Forecast*, *Diabetes Self-Management* or *Diabetes Health*.

- Visit the following websites for timely and accurate diabetes information:

  - Joslin Diabetes Center: www.joslin.org
  - American Diabetes Association: www.diabetes.org
  - American Dietetic Association: www.eatright.org
  - American Association of Diabetes Educators: www.diabeteseducator.org
  - Juvenile Diabetes Research Foundation: www.jdrf.org
  - Centers for Disease Control and Prevention: www.cdc.gov
  - National Diabetes Information Clearinghouse: www.diabetes.niddk.nih.gov
  - National Diabetes Education Program: www.ndep.nih.gov
  - International Diabetes Foundation: www.idf.org
  - Diabetes Self-Management: www.diabetesselfmanagement.com
  - DLife: www.dlife.com

- There are other ways to help you stay healthy with diabetes. For example, you might decide to join the local YMCA, or sign up for a commercial weight-loss program. Many of the diabetes Web sites listed above provide forums and blogs for you and others to share ideas and tips and to problem-solve. There are even games on social media sites such as Facebook that can help you with your diabetes, too. Take advantage of all that's out there.

- There are websites and other sources of diabetes information that may not be so reliable or accurate. If something sounds too good to be true, chances are, it is! Any time that you're unsure about any kind of health information, talk to your provider or diabetes educator for guidance.

Notes and Reminders

Notes and Reminders